The Pharmacist's Guide to Antimicrobial Therapy and Stewardship

Sarah M. Wieczorkiewicz, PharmD, BCPS (AQ-ID)
Clinical Pharmacist, Infectious Diseases
Director, PGY-1 Pharmacy Residency Program
Advocate Lutheran General Hospital
Park Ridge, Illinois

Carrie A. Sincak, PharmD, BCPS, FASHP
Assistant Dean for Clinical Affairs
Professor of Pharmacy Practice
Midwestern University Chicago College of Pharmacy
Downers Grove, Illinois

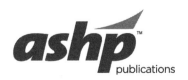

Any correspondence regarding this publication should be sent to the publisher, American Society of Health-System Pharmacists, 7272 Wisconsin Avenue, Bethesda, MD 20814, attention: Special Publishing.

The information presented herein reflects the opinions of the contributors and advisors. It should not be interpreted as an official policy of ASHP or as an endorsement of any product.

Because of ongoing research and improvements in technology, the information and its applications contained in this text are constantly evolving and are subject to the professional judgment and interpretation of the practitioner due to the uniqueness of a clinical situation. The editors and ASHP have made reasonable efforts to ensure the accuracy and appropriateness of the information presented in this document. However, any user of this information is advised that the editors and ASHP are not responsible for the continued currency of the information, for any errors or omissions, and/or for any consequences arising from the use of the information in the document in any and all practice settings. Any reader of this document is cautioned that ASHP makes no representation, guarantee, or warranty, express or implied, as to the accuracy and appropriateness of the information contained in this document and specifically disclaims any liability to any party for the accuracy and/or completeness of the material or for any damages arising out of the use or non-use of any of the information contained in this document.

Director, Special Publishing: Jack Bruggeman
Editorial Project Manager: Ruth Bloom
Production Manager: Johnna Hershey
Cover Design: Carol Barrer

Library of Congress Cataloging-in-Publication Data

Wieczorkiewicz, Sarah M., author.
 The pharmacist's guide to antimicrobial therapy and stewardship / Sarah M. Wieczorkiewicz, Carrie A. Sincak.
  p. ; cm.
 Includes bibliographical references and index.
 ISBN 978-1-58528-519-8 (alk. paper)
 I. Sincak, Carrie A., author. II. American Society of Health-System Pharmacists, issuing body. III. Title.
 [DNLM: 1. Anti-Infective Agents—therapeutic use—Practice Guideline. 2. Anti-Infective Agents—pharmacology—Practice Guideline. 3. Infection—diagnosis—Practice Guideline. 4. Infection—drug therapy—Practice Guideline. 5. Pharmacists—Practice Guideline. QV 250]
 RM267
 615.7'92—dc23
                                                                          2015033760

ISBN: 978-1-58528-519-8

10 9 8 7 6 5 4 3 2 1

Dedication

This guide is dedicated to our students and residents who continue to inspire us to be better preceptors and clinicians for our patients.

~SW and CS

For my late Dad, who continuously instructed, modeled, coached, and facilitated the value of hard work. He was the ultimate preceptor.

~SW

Contents

Preface

In the ever-changing practice of medicine, there is an abundance of gray area and very little in terms of black and white decision-making, especially within the specialty of infectious diseases (ID). As preceptors and practicing clinicians, we have seen many providers struggle with the gray area of ID management. The primary purpose of this point-of-care guide is to provide a simplified, comprehensive, and quick reference on the most commonly encountered ID states and anti-infectives to assist with how to evaluate and manage patients with suspected or confirmed infection. This text begins with the basics of how to assess these patients and progresses to the more challenging recommendations for antimicrobial therapy with subsequent antimicrobial stewardship-related interventions. This reference is specifically designed for the non-ID specialist pharmacists, pharmacy residents, and student pharmacists, although it contains information that would be helpful to all healthcare personnel providing direct patient care in various settings (i.e., acute care, long-term care, ambulatory care). Content may be reviewed generally to gather information on overall key concepts or for specific disease state or drug-specific information.

Organization and Content
The content is separated into five parts describing a general approach for ID patient assessment, treatment, monitoring, and antimicrobial stewardship.

Part I: How to Evaluate a Potentially Infected Patient
This section provides a step-wise approach for the evaluation of a patient with a suspected or confirmed infection and lays the foundation for the remainder of the reference. It contains a flow chart illustrating the steps to take throughout the patient evaluation process. In the first step, clinicians determine whether a confirmed infection is present or absent based on specific subjective and objective data. Also included is how to differentiate between colonization, contamination, and infection based on symptomatology and the variety of culture data available for the patient. Information on the development and interpretation of an antibiogram as well as details about the most clinically significant microorganisms is included. The next subsection covers healthcare-associated risk factors that predispose patients for infection or colonization with multidrug-resistant organisms.

Part II: What Is the Suspected Source of Infection and What Organisms Are Typically Associated with Infection at This Site?
This section includes information about the most commonly encountered ID listed in tabular format that include the following: definition (e.g., diagnostic criteria, clinical presentation, symptoms), most common offending pathogens, treatment and monitoring recommendations (i.e., empiric and definitive with comments on de-escalation when applicable), and duration of therapy. Clinical pearls and comments may also be found throughout this section.

Part III: What Anti-Infectives Provide Adequate Coverage for the Suspected Infection?

This section includes information about antifungals, antimicrobials, and antivirals by drug class in tabular format so as to provide the reader with the quick ability to compare within the class. Drug information includes generic names, mechanism of action, spectrum of activity (including general comparisons), FDA- and non-FDA-approved indications, pharmacodynamics, pharmacokinetics, distribution, the most pertinent adverse effects and drug interactions, common doses, monitoring requirements, resistance mechanisms, and specific comments about each agent.

Part IV: What Patient- or Disease State-Specific Factors Affect Your Decision?

This section focuses on information regarding antimicrobial allergies and ways to approach patients, a renal dose adjustment chart, antimicrobial pharmacodynamics definitions and key concepts, and antimicrobial pharmacokinetics with dosing and monitoring recommendations for vancomycin and aminoglycosides.

Part V: What Antimicrobial Stewardship Interventions Can Be Made on Reassessment and What Needs to Be Monitored?

The last section focuses on the basics of antimicrobial stewardship (AMS), including where to start with the development of an AMS team and how to maintain the program. It begins with the rationale for AMS and describes content on the following: unintended consequences of antimicrobial misuse or overuse, purpose and goals of AMS, key AMS stakeholders and their role in AMS initiatives, description of specific AMS interventions, information on how to monitor and report AMS data, a general approach to the delivery of educational efforts, and critical references to utilize.

Origins of Our Book

The idea for this point-of-care guide originated from self-developed drug tables and general ID information created as a reference to utilize throughout my ID fellowship training that was inspired by Carrie's lectures in pharmacy school. This information was a quick reference to utilize while on rounds. Subsequently, when asked to deliver a "Bugs and Drugs" overview to fourth-year pharmacy students prior to the start of rotations, these tables served as the framework for the lecture. Since this time, it is noted that worn-out copies of these tables continue to circulate. As a result, the idea for sharing this information as a guide was conceived.

We hope this reference will serve as a concise, step-by-step guide to enhance students', residents', and pharmacists' knowledge and application of ID to positively impact the care they provide their patients, and to become an increasing part of their anti-infective decision-making.

Sarah M. Wieczorkiewicz
Carrie A. Sincak
January 2016

Acknowledgments

We are deeply indebted to Robin Coleman for his persistence on the publication of our vision and Ruth Bloom for her exceptional patience, diligence, and attention to detail on this project. Her firm guidance helped us to remain on task. We would also like to thank Johnna Hershey (Production) and the support staff in Special Publishing and Marketing at the American Society of Health-System Pharmacists for their assistance throughout the process.

We would be remiss not to acknowledge our spouses, Jeff and Keith, and children, Madelyn, Francesca, Henry, and Reagan, for their support, love, and understanding as we worked on this project.

Abbreviations

aBW	adjusted body weight
AECB	acute exacerbations of chronic bronchitis
AF	atrial fibrillation
AG	aminoglycoside
ALT	alanine aminotransferase
AMS	antimicrobial stewardship
ANC	absolute neutrophil count
ARDS	acute respiratory distress syndrome
AST	aspartate aminotransferase
AUC	area under the curve
AUC/MIC	area under the concentration time curve to minimum inhibitory concentration ratio
BID	twice a day
BP	blood pressure
BSI	bloodstream infections
CA-MRSA	community-acquired methicillin-resistant *Staphylococcus aureus*
CAP	community-acquired pneumonia
CAPD	continuous ambulatory peritoneal dialysis
CAVH	continuous arteriovenous hemofiltration
CBC	complete blood count
CF	cystic fibrosis
CFU	colony forming unit
CLSI	Clinical Laboratory Standards Institute
C_{max}/MIC	maximum drug concentration to minimum inhibitory concentration ratio
CMV	cytomegalovirus
CNS	central nervous system
COPD	chronic obstructive pulmonary disease
CrCl	creatinine clearance
CRE	carbapenem-resistant *Enterobacteriaceae*
CSF	cerebrospinal fluid
CT	computed tomography scan
CV	cardiovascular
CVP	central venous pressure
CVVH	continuous veno-venous hemofiltration
DS	double strength
DW	dosing weight

ECHO	echocardiogram (an ultrasound evaluation of the heart)
ED	emergency department
EPS	extrapyramidal symptoms
erm	erythromycin ribosome methylation
ESBL	extended spectrum β lactamase
ET	endotracheal
EtOH	ethanol
FQ	fluoroquinolone
GI	gastrointestinal
GU	genitourinary
HA	headache
HAP	hospital-acquired pneumonia
HCAP	healthcare-associated pneumonia
HD	hemodialysis
Heme	hematology
HGB/HCT	hemoglobin/hematocrit
HSV	herpes simplex virus
Hx	history
IBW	ideal body weight
ICU	intensive care unit
IgE	immunoglobulin E
IgG	immunoglobulin G
IHD	intermittent hemodialysis
IM	intramuscular
INH	isoniazid
IV	intravenous
IVC	inferior vena cava
IVIG	intravenous immunoglobulin
K	potassium
KPC	*Klebsiella pneumoniae* carbapenemase
LFT	liver function test
LRTI	lower respiratory tract infections
MAO	monoamine oxidase
MAP	mean arterial pressure
MBC	minimum bactericidal concentration
MDR	multidrug-resistant
MDRO	multidrug-resistant organism
Mg	magnesium
MIC	minimum inhibitory concentration
MRI	magnetic resonance imaging
MRSA	methicillin-resistant *Staphylococcus aureus*

MRSE	methicillin-resistant *Staphylococcus epidermidis*
MSSA	methicillin-susceptible *Staphylococcus aureus*
MSSE	methicillin-susceptible *Staphylococcus epidermidis*
Na	sodium
NDA	new drug application
NRTIs	nucleoside reverse transcriptase inhibitors
P	desired peak
PABA	para-aminobenzoic acid
PAE	post-antibiotic effect
PCN	penicillin
PD	pharmacodynamics
PEG	percutaneous endoscopic gastrostomy
PID	pelvic inflammatory disease
PJP	*Pneumocystis jeroveci*
PN	parenteral nutrition
PO	oral
PO_4	phosphorus
PPE	personal protective equipment
PRBC	packed red blood cells
Q	every
Qnr	quinolone-resistant
QOD	every other day
RBCs	red blood cells
RVR	rapid ventricular response
Rxn	reaction
SBP	systolic blood pressure
SCr	serum creatinine
$Scvo_2$	central venous oxygen saturation
SMX-TMP	sulfamethoxazole/trimethoprim
SSTI	skin and soft tissue infection
T > MIC	time above minimum inhibitory concentration
TEE	transthoracic endoscopic echocardiogram
TEN	toxic epidermal necrolysis
TIW	three times per week
TMP/SMX	trimethoprim/sulfamethoxazole
TSH	thyroid stimulating hormone
TTE	transthoracic transesophageal echocardiogram
URTI	upper respiratory tract infection
UTI	urinary tract infection

VAP	ventilator-associated pneumonia
Vd	population volume of distribution estimate
VISA	vancomycin-intermediate *Staphylococcus aureus*
VRE	vancomycin-resistant *Entercoccus*
VRSA	vancomycin-resistant *Staphylococcus aureus*
VZV	varicella zoster virus
WBCs	white blood cells

PART I

How to Evaluate
a Potentially
Infected Patient

I.1   IS THE PATIENT INFECTED?

One of the most challenging issues in infectious diseases is determining whether the cause of the patient's symptoms is as a direct result of an infection or another non-infectious etiology such as malignancy, emboli, autoimmune diseases, or drug-related. See table below for specific examples.

Etiologies That May Mimic Infection	Symptoms Similar to Infection
Malignancy	• Fever • Night sweats • Lymphadenopathy • Leukocytosis (especially leukemia) • Tumor may resemble abscess
Emboli	• Fever • Swelling • Erythema • Pain • Shortness of breath
Autoimmune disease	• Swelling • Erythema • Pain • Diarrhea, abdominal pain, etc. associated with some autoimmune diseases such as Crohn's disease and ulcerative colitis may resemble *Clostridium difficile* infection • Increased non-specific inflammatory markers such as ESR, CRP
Corticosteroids	• May mimic or mask infection • Mimic: cause a temporary leukocytosis with high doses, no left shift (demargination) • Mask: potent anti-inflammatory effect decreases natural inflammatory reaction to infection and ablates febrile response

Drug fever	• In general, patients who do not usually have rigors will not exhibit other signs and symptoms of infection
	• Usually these patients are unaware of fever
	• Often but not always chronic, non-spiking nature of temperature
	• Time of onset not usually helpful (can occur days to weeks after the initiation of the drug)
	• Usually subsides 72–96 hours after cessation of the offending agent
	• Most common agents associated with drug fever:
	  ○ Anticonvulsants (e.g., carbamazepine, phenytoin, phenobarbital, primidone)
	  ○ Minocycline
	  ○ Other antimicrobials (e.g., β-lactams, sulfonamides, nitrofurantoin)
	  ○ Allopurinol

Once the decision has been made that an infection is present, clinicians can then begin to think about the potential source of infection based on subjective and objective evidence and decide on appropriate therapy. The flow chart on next page describes the steps to take when evaluating patients with suspected or confirmed infection.

How to Evaluate a Potentially Infected Patient

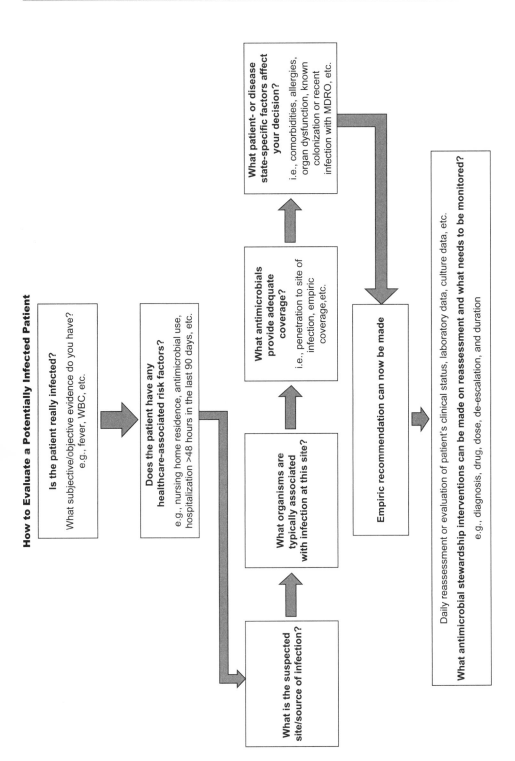

Is the patient really infected?
What subjective/objective evidence do you have?
e.g., fever, WBC, etc.

Does the patient have any healthcare-associated risk factors?
e.g., nursing home residence, antimicrobial use, hospitalization >48 hours in the last 90 days, etc.

What is the suspected site/source of infection?

What organisms are typically associated with infection at this site?

What antimicrobials provide adequate coverage?
i.e., penetration to site of infection, empiric coverage, etc.

What patient- or disease state-specific factors affect your decision?
i.e., comorbidities, allergies, organ dysfunction, known colonization or recent infection with MDRO, etc.

Empiric recommendation can now be made

Daily reassessment or evaluation of patient's clinical status, laboratory data, culture data, etc.
What antimicrobial stewardship interventions can be made on reassessment and what needs to be monitored?
e.g., diagnosis, drug, dose, de-escalation, and duration

HOW TO EVALUATE A PATIENT WITH A POTENTIAL INFECTIOUS DISEASE STATE

Question 1: Is the patient really infected? Collect all subjective and objective data to support or refute possibility of infection.

Question 2: Does the patient have any healthcare-associated risk factors? If so, consider how many risk factors, type of risk, etc.

Question 3: What is the suspected site/source of infection? Use information from above to justify rationale.

Question 4: What organisms are typically associated with infection at this site (e.g., normal flora *versus* colonization)?

Question 5: What anti-infectives will provide adequate coverage and will reach the site of infection?

Question 6: What patient- or disease state-specific factors affect your decision?

Question 7: Once more data become available (usually within 48–72 hours but should be reassessed daily) such as patient's clinical status, laboratory data, culture data, etc., what antimicrobial stewardship interventions can be made on reassessment and what needs to be monitored (e.g., diagnosis, drug, dose, de-escalation, duration)?

EXAMPLE

MR is an 82-yo-female who presents to the ED from an extended-care facility (ECF) with fever, shortness of breath, and cough for the past 24 hours. She is currently at the ECF for rehabilitation status post hip replacement surgery eight days ago. Prior to the hip replacement surgery, she was independent with her ADLs and lived alone at home.

Allergies: NKA

PMH: Hypertension, hyperlipidemia, osteoarthritis

SH: + tobacco (quit 10 years ago, 1ppd × 30 years), + alcohol (1 glass of wine 3–4 nights per week), – illicits

Vitals: T: 101.3°F, BP: 101/67, HR: 88, RR: 19, SpO_2: 93–95%

Height: 62″   **Weight:** 74 kg

Labs:

$$15.1 \diagup \dfrac{14.2}{41.7} \diagdown 259 \qquad \dfrac{139 \mid 104 \mid 18}{3.8 \mid 25 \mid 1.01} \diagdown 96$$

CXR: + left lower lobe infiltrate

UA: negative

Sputum culture: pending

Rapid influenza: negative

Patient is hemodynamically stable and is being admitted to the general medicine floor.

Question 1:   Is the patient really infected? List all subjective and objective data to support or refute possibility of infection.
Yes, the patient is infected.
Subjective – fever at long-term care facility, shortness of breath, and cough
Objective – T 101.3°F, SpO$_2$ 93–95%, WBC 15.1, + infiltrate on CXR

Question 2:   Does the patient have any healthcare-associated risk factors? If so, consider how many risk factors, type of risk, etc.
Extended care facility

Question 3:   What is the suspected site/source of infection? Use information from above to justify rationale.
Lung—cough, shortness of breath, infiltrate

Question 4:   What organisms are typically associated with infection at this site (e.g., normal flora *versus* colonization)?
Gram −: Escherichia coli, Klebsiella pneumoniae, Enterobacter spp. *Proteus* spp.,
Serratia marcescens, Pseudomonas aeruginosa, Acinetobacter spp.
Gram +: +/− MRSA

Question 5:   What anti-infectives will provide adequate coverage and will reach the site of infection?
Gram – coverage: anti-pseudomonal β-lactam (e.g., piperacillin/tazobactam, cefepime, ceftazidime, meropenem, imipenem/cilastatin, or doripenem), monobactam (e.g., aztreonam), +/− fluoroquinolone (e.g., ciprofloxacin or levofloxacin) or aminoglycoside (e.g., gentamicin, tobramycin, or amikacin)
Gram + coverage: vancomycin or linezolid

Question 6:   What patient- or disease state-specific factors affect your decision (e.g., patient weight, renal and hepatic function, comorbidities, allergies, etc.)?
IBW: 50.1 kg
Actual BW: 72 kg
Adjusted BW: 58.9 kg
Estimated CrCl: 39.9 mL/min

What is the final empiric recommendation including anticipated duration of anti-infective therapy and monitoring parameters?

- *Piperacillin/tazobactam 3.375 g Q8h over 4 hours (extended infusion): reassess every day and monitor renal function, improvement in clinical status, resolution in clinical signs and symptoms; assess sputum culture.*
- *She is hemodynamically stable with relatively few risk factors and is admitted to the general medicine floor. She is not likely to have MRSA pneumonia.*
- *Would not treat with vancomycin or linezolid. Treatment for HCAP should not exceed 7–8 days unless infected with a nonfermenting gram negative bacilli.*

Question 7:   Once more data become available (i.e., patient's clinical status, laboratory data, culture data, etc.): What antimicrobial stewardship interventions can be made on reassessment and what needs to be monitored (e.g., diagnosis, drug, dose, de-escalation, duration)?
What is the final recommendation including duration of anti-infective therapy and monitoring parameters?

- *Treatment for HCAP should not exceed 7 to 8 days unless infected with a nonfermenting gram negative bacilli (e.g., Pseudomonas aeruginosa, Acinetobacter spp.).*
- *Monitor renal function, clinical status, signs and symptoms of infection resolution (i.e., cough, fever, shortness of breath, etc.), and for adverse effects.*
- *May consider de-escalation of therapy once sputum culture data are available. If no positive cultures as is common in pneumonia, may consider de-escalation to an oral fluoroquinolone such as ciprofloxacin or levofloxacin to complete therapy.*

WHEN TO TREAT, WHEN NOT TO TREAT—THAT IS A GOOD QUESTION

The following information provides guidance on how to differentiate between colonization, contamination, and infection; interpret culture data; and decipher institutional antibiogram data. These data should be considered when deciding if a patient has an infection or another non-infectious source of symptoms.

Differentiation between Colonization, Contamination, and Infection

Colonization: The presence of microorganisms without host inflammatory response.
Contamination: The presence of microorganisms typically acquired during acquisition or processing of host specimens without evidence of host inflammatory response.
Infection: The presence of one or more microorganisms with host inflammatory response.

Sterile anatomical sites: Sites that are normally sterile include CSF, blood, lungs, urinary tract, and biliary tract. If microorganisms are cultured from these sites, they may likely be pathogenic; however, they still sometimes represent contamination or colonization. Clinical correlation is essential for interpretation.

Non-Sterile anatomical sites: Sites that are normally non-sterile include sputum, pus, skin swabs, GI tract, and vagina. It is expected that microorganisms will grow in specimens from non-sterile sites. For interpretation, consider whether the identified microorganisms correlate to the clinical syndrome.

Colonization/Contamination	Infection
• Normal white count, no left shift (increased bands)	• WBCs elevated or decreased with left shift • WBC may be decreased in overwhelming sepsis and may be unchanged in indolent or subacute infection (e.g., abscess, endocarditis)
• Not typically associated with WBCs	• WBCs often present
• Normothermia	• Hyperthermia or hypothermia
• Usually not associated with heavy growth of pathogen on Gram stain	• More often associated with heavy growth of pathogen on a Gram stain
• Not associated with other signs of an infection	• Usually associated with other signs of an infection (see below)

Clinical, Laboratory, and Radiographic Signs of Infection	
CLINICAL	
Localized	Diarrhea, nausea, vomiting, abdominal distention
	Dysuria, frequency, urgency (UTI)
	Headache, stiff neck, photophobia, unexplained seizures (meningitis)
	Pain and inflammation at site of infection—erythema, swelling, warmth, wound, skin lesion, abscess
	Purulent discharge (wound, vaginal, urethral)
	Sputum production and cough (pneumonia)
	Chills, rigors
Systemic	Hypo- or hyperthermia
	Malaise
	Tachycardia
	Tachypnea
	Hypotension
	Hypoxemia, acidosis/alkalosis
	Mental status changes (especially in elderly patients)
	Weakness
LABORATORY	
Elevated erythrocyte sedimentation rate (ESR), C-reactive protein (CRP), or procalcitonin (PCT)	
Elevated or depressed white blood cell count—peripherally or at the site of infection	
Elevated lactate	
Increased immature neutrophils (bands) in the WBC differential (left shift)	
Positive antigen test or antibody titers	
Positive Gram stain and/or culture from site of infection (always evaluate patient's clinical status and symptomatology)	
RADIOGRAPHIC	
Bone x-ray or MRI with periosteal elevation or bony destruction in patients with osteomyelitis	
Chest x-ray or CT with consolidation, infiltrate, effusion, or cavitary nodules in patients with lung infections	
Abdominal ultrasound or CT with evidence of perforation or abscess	
ECHO with vegetations (endocarditis)	
Head CT/MRI—ring enhancing lesions in patients with brain abscesses	

HOW TO INTERPRET CULTURE DATA

Culture Type*	Factors to Consider	Is Your Patient Infected?
Blood	• Contamination occurs frequently • Number of samples collected (sets) are extremely important (i.e., should be two sets from two separate sites at two different times) **False-positives:** • Bacterial growth first occurs after 72 hours of incubation • If common skin commensals present in multiple blood cultures obtained by independent venipuncture, consider presence of prosthetic material and subjective/objective patient data • Only one set positive out of two or more (also consider same site versus different sites) • *Propionibacterium acnes, Corynebacterium* spp., *Bacillus* spp., or Coagulase-negative *Staphylococcus* (*Staphylococcus epidermidis*) in patients without prosthetic material	If common colonizing organism present, look for corresponding subjective and objective data such as leukocytosis, left shift, fever/chills, risk factors If patients have prosthetic material such as heart valves or devices, common skin commensals require careful assessment as they may be pathogenic
	The following organisms are almost always significant and require treatment regardless of number positive: • *Enterococcus* spp. • Gram negative organisms • Group A *Streptococcus* and most other *Streptococcus* spp. • *S. aureus* • Yeast (e.g., *Candida* spp.)	
Sputum	• Colonization also occurs frequently in patients who are chronically ill with chronic tracheostomies or those who are chronically ventilated • Colonization occurs frequently due to most cultures representing upper airway secretions as opposed to actual sputum • Mixed flora may grow on Gram stain in the absence of bacterial infection • Organism concentrations and clinical correlations are essential • Shows presence of squamous epithelial cells > 10 = contaminated • Is reported in a quantitative manner, e.g., 1+ to 4+ or rare, few, moderate, abundant • Some organisms are almost never considered pulmonary pathogens such as Coagulase-negative *Staphylococcus, Enterococcus,* gram + bacilli (except *Nocardia* spp.), certain *Streptococcus* spp. (except *pneumoniae, agalactiae, pyogenes*, and *anginosus*), and *Candida* spp. • True pathogens usually present in at least 3+ or moderate amount	Regardless of the organisms identified, it is absolutely essential to evaluate and assess the subjective and objective data to support or refute active infection due to incidence of frequent colonization (e.g., leukocytosis, left shift, fever/chills, cough, shortness of breath, respiratory rate, oxygen saturations, increased purulent secretions, increased suctioning requirements in tracheostomy/ventilated patients, etc.)

Culture Type*	Factors to Consider	Is Your Patient Infected?
Urinalysis	**Positive culture defined as the following:** • >10^5 CFU (organism) • ≥ 10,000 leukocytes/mL • Positive nitrites (indicates presence of *Enterobacteriaceae*) • Positive leukocyte esterase	Asymptomatic bacteriuria should not be treated unless the patient is pregnant or is undergoing a GU surgical procedure. Evaluate the patient for presence of subjective and objective findings as well as presence of an indwelling Foley catheter. If Foley catheter present, remove or replace and reculture after 24 hours if symptoms develop.

(continued)

Culture Type*	Factors to Consider					Is Your Patient Infected?
		Normal	Bacterial Meningitis	Viral Meningitis	Fungal Meningitis	
CSF – Lumbar Puncture	Opening pressure	60–200 mm H_2O*	Markedly elevated	Normal (may be slightly elevated but uncommon)	Elevated	Red blood cells in the CSF may indicate a traumatic tap or subarachnoid hemorrhage. If traumatic tap, protein and white blood cell count are falsely elevated. To correct, use the following equations: Protein—subtract 1 mg/dL for every 1,000 RBCs WBC—subtract 1 cell/mm^3 for every 500–1,000 RBCs Glucose can be altered in a variety of conditions. Pay careful attention to serum glucose. Newborns have higher CSF: serum glucose ratios and those with severe hyperglycemia.
	Color	Clear	Cloudy	+/–Cloudy	+/–Cloudy	
	WBC (cells/mm³)	≤5 (≤20 in newborns)	1,000–5,000	100–500	100–500	
	Predominant cell type	70% Lymphocytes	>80% Neutrophils	Lymphocytes	Lymphocytes	
	Glucose	60% of serum glucose	Low	Normal	Low	
	Protein (mg/dL)	20–45 (20–170 in neonates)	Elevated 100–500	Normal (may be slightly elevated)	Elevated	
	Lactate (mg/dL)	10–27	Elevated	Normal	May be elevated	

* Obese patients may have opening pressures up to 250 mmH$_2$O and the range for children <8 years of age is lower (10–100 mmH$_2$O)

* It is best to obtain all cultures prior to administration of anti-infectives; however, anti-infective administration should not be delayed especially in a patient with sepsis.

HOW TO INTERPRET AN ANTIBIOGRAM

What Is an Antibiogram?
- A record usually produced semi-annually or annually of antimicrobial susceptibility for bacterial isolates collected at a hospital or outpatient facility
- Presents a spectrum of susceptibility to antimicrobials that exists among common microorganisms detected by the laboratory
- Must have at least 30 isolates of a specific pathogen to report susceptibilities
- The antibiogram is used to:
  - Assess local susceptibility rates
  - Monitor resistance trends over time
  - Guide selection of empiric antimicrobial treatment
  - Guide decisions about which antimicrobials are included on formularies

Example Antibiogram

Organism	# Isolates Identified	Drug #1	Drug #2	Drug #3
Organism #1	1,450	100%	77%	99%
Organism #2	500	100%	90%	81%
Organism #3	202	100%	63%	70%
Organism #4	2,450	100%	65%	96%

How to Use the Tables
Number of isolates reflects the number of isolates that have yielded positive for colonies of the given organism during the time period assessed.

The percentage (%) reported reflects the total number of isolates susceptible to the antimicrobial.

Organism	# Isolates Identified	Drug #1	Drug #2	Interpretation
Organism #1	1,450	100%	77%	Organism #1 is 100% susceptible to Drug #1 and 77% susceptible to Drug #2

- When testing, data are obtained by broth microdilution, alternative MIC (minimum inhibitory concentration) methods, or disk diffusion testing according to Clinical and Laboratory Standards Institute (CLSI) guidelines.
- This chart will determine if an organism is susceptible, susceptible dose-dependent, intermediate, or resistant to an antimicrobial. Susceptible implies that an infection due to the microorganism may be appropriately treated with the dosage of antimicrobial agent recommended for the infecting species and the site of infection.
  - *Susceptible (S)* = isolates are inhibited by usually achievable concentrations of the antimicrobial when the dosage recommended to treat the site of infection is used.
  - *Susceptible Dose Dependent (S-DD)* = isolates may be susceptible based on antimicrobial dosing (i.e., higher doses, more frequent dosing, or both may be required).
  - *Intermediate (I)* = isolates with MICs that approach usually attainable blood and tissue levels and for which response rates may be lower than susceptible isolates.

○ *Resistant (R)* = isolates are not inhibited by the usually achievable concentrations of the agent with normal dosage schedules and/or demonstrate MICs or zone sizes that fall in the range where resistance mechanisms are likely.
- MIC is the lowest concentration of a drug that will inhibit growth of a microorganism in vitro.
  ○ Lowest MIC on a susceptibility report does not necessarily indicate the best treatment option.
  ○ MICs are specific to each microorganism and antimicrobial.

ANTIBIOGRAM LIMITATIONS

- Antibiograms do not provide syndrome or disease-specific advice.
- There is no distribution of organisms for a given infection.
- It is not helpful in polymicrobial infections or infections empirically treated with more than one agent.
- Current hospital antibiograms do not take into account risk factors that can influence susceptibility (such as presenting living situation).
- They lack external validity and are only applicable to single site.

1.2   CLINICALLY SIGNIFICANT MICROORGANISM BASICS

Organism Type	Specific Organisms		Recommended (R) and Alternative (A) Treatment	Common Types of Related Infections	Comments
Aerobic gram positive cocci in clusters	Staphylococcus	S. aureus			
		MSSA	**R:** Oxacillin, nafcillin, cefazolin **A:** Vancomycin, clindamycin Many additional agents have activity, however, are not preferred as first- or second-line	• Bacteremia • CNS • Endocarditis • Joint infections • Osteomyelitis • PNA • Prosthetic device-related infections • SSTIs	• Virulent • Hearty; grows easily • 20–30% of population colonized with S. aureus • If bacteremia, must rule out endocarditis (20–30% of S. aureus bacteremia) • D-test utilized to detect inducible clindamycin resistance
		CA-MRSA	**R:** TMP-SMX, minocycline/doxycycline, clindamycin (↑resistance) **A:** Vancomycin, oxazolidinones, daptomycin, quinupristin/dalfopristin, ceftaroline, lipoglycopeptides	• PNA • SSTIs	• Especially virulent due to Panton Valentine Leukocidin toxin production; causes tissue necrosis • High risk groups include children, prisoners, MSM, IVDUs • If bacteremia, must rule out endocarditis (20–30% of S. aureus bacteremia) • SSTIs/PNA are the most common; however, same infection types as MSSA are possible • No daptomycin for PNA (inactivated by surfactant) • D-test utilized to detect inducible clindamycin resistance
		HA-MRSA	**R:** Vancomycin	• Bacteremia • Endocarditis	• Virulent • If bacteremia, must rule out endocarditis (20–30% of S. aureus bacteremia)

Organism Type	Specific Organisms		Recommended (R) and Alternative (A) Treatment	Common Types of Related Infections	Comments
Aerobic gram positive cocci in clusters (*Cont'd*)	Staphylococcus	*S. aureus*	HA-MRSA	A: Daptomycin, oxazolidinones, quinupristin/dalfopristin, lipoglycopeptides, ceftaroline, tigecycline	• PNA • PNA, bacteremia, and endocarditis are the most common; however, same infection types as MSSA are possible	• No daptomycin for PNA (inactivated by surfactant)
		S. epidermidis (Coagulase-negative Staphylococcus)		R: Vancomycin +/– rifampin (+ gentamicin for prosthetic valve endocarditis) A: Linezolid, daptomycin, or lipoglycopeptides +/– rifampin Oxacillin, nafcillin may be used if susceptible (>75–80% resistant); also if MRSE, cefazolin, fluoroquinolones, clindamycin, or TMP-SMX may be considered based on susceptibilities	• Bacteremia • Endocarditis • Other prosthetic device/material-related infections	• Frequent contaminant found on the skin and mucous membranes • Consider number of positive cultures (≥2 for blood) and patient risk factors • Oftentimes hospital-acquired • Commonly associated with prosthetic materials and biofilm production
		S. lugdunesis (Coagulase-negative Staphylococcus)		R: Oxacillin, nafcillin, or penicillin G A: First-generation cephalosporins, vancomycin	• Bacteremia • Endocarditis • Other prosthetic device/material-related infections	• Virulent • Involved in severe infections • More common in immuno-compromised patients • More susceptible to oxacillin, nafcillin than S. *epidermidis*
Aerobic gram positive cocci in pairs and chains	Streptococcus	*S. pyogenes* (Group A; β-hemolytic)		R: Penicillin G + clindamycin (must use combination in severe infections; clindamycin halts toxin production)	• SSTIs • Pharyngitis "Strep throat"	• ~5% adults and 15–20% school-age children colonized (pharynx)

Category	Organism	Treatment	Infections	Notes
Aerobic gram positive cocci in pairs and chains (Cont'd) — Streptococcus		A: Penicillin or clindamycin alone		• Can cause severe, life-threatening infections including toxic shock syndrome, due to a multitude of virulence factors (e.g., M proteins, pyrogenic exotoxins, etc.) • Complications include rheumatic fever
	S. agalactiae (Group B)	R: Penicillin G +/– gentamicin (for serious infections add gentamicin) A: Vancomycin, clindamycin (some strains resistant)	• Bacteremia/endocarditis (especially in immuno-compromised patients) • Chorioamnionitis • Neonatal sepsis and meningitis • Septic arthritis • SSTIs • UTIs (young sexually-active females or adults >65)	• Number one cause of neonatal morbidity and mortality
	S. bovis (Group D)	R: Penicillin G +/– gentamicin A: Clindamycin (some strains resistant)	• Bacteremia • Endocarditis	• Normal colonizer of the GI tract • Strongly associated with colonic malignancy (patients should always be evaluated)
	S. pneumoniae	R: Penicillin G or amoxicillin for penicillin susceptible Ceftriaxone, moxifloxacin, levofloxacin, amoxicillin (high dose), linezolid, vancomycin for penicillin resistant A: Second- and third-generation cephalosporins, clindamycin, ceftaroline, azithromycin	• PNA • Sinusitis • Meningitis • Otitis media • COPD/chronic bronchitis exacerbations • Bacteremia	• Nasopharynx colonizer • Often cause of PNA immediately after recent influenza • If meningitis, higher doses required

(continued)

Organism Type	Specific Organisms	Recommended (R) and Alternative (A) Treatment	Common Types of Related Infections	Comments
Aerobic gram positive cocci in pairs and chains *(Cont'd)*	**Strepto- coccus** Viridans group Streptococci	**R:** Penicillin G +/− gentamicin, ceftriaxone **A:** Vancomycin Tetracyclines, macrolides, and clindamycin ↑resistance	• Bacteremia (may be contaminant) • Dental infections • Endocarditis	• Normal oral and GI flora
	Entero- coccus *E. faecalis*	**R:** Ampicillin (if susceptible) or vancomycin +/− gentamicin (endocarditis) Ceftriaxone + ampicillin for endocarditis **A:** Linezolid, daptomycin	• Bacteremia • Endocarditis • Intra-abdominal • Meningitis (with risk factors such as neuro-surgery, head trauma, etc.) • UTIs	• *E. faecalis* not as virulent • Normal GI and female GU tract flora • Resistance seen with these organisms (especially VRE) • Chronically ill or nursing home residents more likely to be colonized with VRE
	E. faecium	**R:** Vancomycin, ampicillin (if susceptible) **A:** Linezolid, daptomycin, quin-upristin/dalfopristin		
Aerobic gram positive bacilli (rods)	**Diphther-oids** *Corynebacterium*	**R:** Vancomycin +/− aminoglycoside **A:** Penicillin + aminoglycoside	• Prosthetic material-related infections	• Oftentimes contaminant
	Propionibacterium acnes	**R:** Penicillin G **A:** Clindamycin, vancomycin, daptomycin, linezolid <u>For acne:</u> tetracycline, minocycline, doxycycline, erythromycin, TMP-SMX	• Acne • CNS infections • Endocarditis • Osteomyelitis	• Oftentimes contaminant • Normal skin, nasopharynx, and GI/GU flora • Device-related infections (difficult to differentiate between contaminant and pathogen) • Slow-growing organism

Aerobic gram positive bacilli (rods) (Cont'd)	Diphtheroids	Listeria monocytogenes	P: Ampicillin +/– gentamicin for synergy A: SMP-TMX	• Meningitis (patients > 50 y/o, neonates, and immunocompromised) • Sepsis	• Hardy pathogen and can withstand cold, moist environment • Foodborne pathogen (in high risk groups such as elderly, pregnancy, immunocompromised)—unpasteurized dairy, deli meats, etc.
Aerobic and facultative anaerobic gram negative rods (bacilli)	Enterobacteriaceae	Escherichia coli	R: TMP-SMX (↑resistance), FQ (↑resistance), ceftriaxone A: Cephalosporins, piperacillin/tazobactam, carbapenems, AG, tigecycline, aztreonam Also effective for UTIs (non-systemic) fosfomycin, nitrofurantoin; do not use moxifloxacin for UTIs	• Bacteremia • CNS infections • GU infections • Intra-abdominal infections • PNA • SSTIs • Traveler's diarrhea • UTIs	• Normal GI tract flora • ESBL producer (incidence increasing) • Susceptibilities should guide therapy
		Klebsiella pneumoniae	R: Cefepime, piperacillin/tazobactam, ceftazidime, AG, FQ, carbapenems A: Tigecycline, colistin Treatment depends on the site of infection and susceptibility	• CNS infections • Intra-abdominal infections • PNA • UTIs	• ESBL producer, plasmid-mediated • Many CRE/KPC producers (consider colistin, tigecycline) • Susceptibilities should guide therapy
		Proteus mirabilis	R: Ciprofloxacin, levofloxacin, ceftriaxone, cefepime, piperacillin/tazobactam A: Carbapenems	• Bacteremia • Intra-abdominal infections • PNA • SSTIs • UTIs	• Organism splits urea with subsequent elevation in urinary pH • Susceptibilities should guide therapy

(continued)

Organism Type	Specific Organisms	Recommended (R) and Alternative (A) Treatment	Common Types of Related Infections	Comments
Aerobic and facultative anaerobic gram negative rods (bacilli) (*Cont'd*)	Enterobacteriaceae			
	Acinetobacter	R: Imipenem/cilastatin, meropenem, ampicillin/sulbactam (high dose)—used for the sulbactam component, colistin, tigecycline, amikacin A: Other AG, minocycline, rifampin, polymixin B	• PNA • Wounds • Bacteremia • May cause numerous infections in immuno-compromised	• Usually multidrug resistant (resistant to: all penicillins, cephalosporins, aztreonam, AG, FQ, and +/− carbapenems) • Can colonize respiratory tract • May require combination therapy (e.g., carbapenem + colistin, carbapenem + sulbactam, tigecycline + carbapenem or colistin) • Susceptibilities should guide therapy
	Shigella dysenteriae	R: FQ, azithromycin A: Ceftriaxone, TMP-SMX (if susceptible)	• Gastroenteritis	• Usually community acquired and seen in recent travelers • Treat all cases with antimicrobials • Replace fluid losses
	Salmonella typhi	R: Ceftriaxone, cefixime A: Ciprofloxacin (if susceptible)	• Gastroenteritis • Typhoid fever	• Usually community acquired • Usually in developing countries or travelers who recently returned from endemic areas • High fevers typical; diarrhea not common • Complications: septic/reactive arthritis, endocarditis, meningitis, osteomyelitis, etc.
	Salmonella spp. (Non typhoid)	Usually self-limiting If serious infection: R: Ceftriaxone A: Ciprofloxacin (if susceptible)	• Gastroenteritis	• Symptoms may resolve and then recur • Can result in chronic colonization

		Organism	Agents (R: recommended / A: alternative)	Infections	Notes
Aerobic and facultative anaerobic gram negative rods (bacilli) (Cont'd)	Enterobacteriaceae	*Morganella morganii*	R: Cefotaxime, ceftriaxone, amoxicillin/clavulanate, second- and third-generation cephalosporins (oral) A: FQ, ampicillin (if susceptible and β-lactamase negative)	• URI	• Usually community acquired
		Citrobacter spp.	R: Cefepime, carbapenem A: FQ, TMP-SMX, AG	• May cause numerous types of infections especially in immunocompromised (UTIs, PNA, bacteremia, etc.)	• Inducible β-lactamases • Oftentimes MDR • Cefepime may develop resistance while on therapy • Susceptibility should guide therapy
		Enterobacter	R: Cefepime, carbapenem A: FQ, AG		• Typically hospital-acquired infections • Avoid FQs as empiric monotherapy in critically ill patients
		Serratia marsecens	R: Cefepime, carbapenems, ciprofloxacin, levofloxacin, AG A: Susceptibility should guide therapy		
		Providencia stuartii	R: Ciprofloxacin, levofloxacin, piperacillin/tazobactam A: Carbapenems, AG, TMP-SMX	• Bacteremia • Pneumonia • Prostatitis • UTIs (usually catheter-associated)	• Avoid cephalosporins • Susceptibilities should guide therapy
	Pseudomonads	*Pseudomonas aeruginosa*	R: Meropenem, doripenem, imipenem/cilastatin, cefepime, ceftazidime, piperacillin/tazobactam A: FQ, colistin, AG, aztreonam, ceftazidime/avibactam, ceftolozane/tazobactam	• May cause numerous infections in immunocompromised (SSTIs, UTIs, PNA)	• Oftentimes MDR • Consider combination empiric therapy in critically ill patients with a high risk for mortality • Susceptibilities should guide therapy

(continued)

Organism Type	Specific Organisms	Recommended (R) and Alternative (A) Treatment	Common Types of Related Infections	Comments
Aerobic and facultative anaerobic gram negative rods (bacilli) (Cont'd)	**Pseudomonads** *Stenotrophomonas maltophilia*	R: TMP-SMX, FQs A: Minocycline, tigecycline, ceftazidime	• May cause numerous infections in immuno-compromised (PNA, SSTIs, bacteremia)	• TMP-SMX 15–20 mg/kg is the drug of choice • May be a respiratory tract colonizer in chronically ventilated patients • Significant and requires treatment when cultured from blood
	Burkholdaria cepacia	R: Ceftazidime, carbapenems (no ertapenem), minocycline A: TMP-SMX, ciprofloxacin	• May cause numerous infections in immuno-compromised (PNA, bacteremia, SSTIs, endocarditis) and cystic fibrosis (CF) exacerbations	• Susceptibilities should guide therapy • Negative prognostic indicator for CF patients
	Coccobacilli *Haemophilus influenzae*	R: Cefotaxime, ceftriaxone, amoxicillin/clavulanate, second- and third-generation cephalosporins (oral) A: FQ, ampicillin (if susceptible and β-lactamase negative), macrolides	• Meningitis • PNA • URIs	• Use cefotaxime or ceftriaxone if meningitis, epiglottitis, or other severe, life-threatening illness
	Bordetella pertussis	R: Macrolides A: TMP/SMX	• Whooping cough	
Aerobic gram negative cocci	*Moraxella catarrhalis*	R: Amoxicillin/clavulanate, second- and third-generation cephalosporins (oral), TMP-SMX A: Macrolides, doxycycline, FQ	• PNA • URIs	

Category	Organism	Treatment	Diseases	Notes
Aerobic gram negative cocci (*Contd*)	*Neisseria gonnorrheae*	R: Ceftriaxone, cefixime PLUS azithromycin	• Cervicitis • Conjunctivitis • Endometritis • Epididymitis • PID • Urethritis	• Extremely virulent and virtually pan-resistant in some parts of the world • FQ resistant rates are high; avoid use • Must treat for concomitant chlamydia
	Neisseria meningitidis	R: Ceftriaxone, cefotaxime A: Meropenem	• Bacteremia • Meningitis	• Vaccine available
Anaerobic gram positive rods (bacilli)	*Clostridium botulinum*	Botulinum immunoglobulin may be required in some patients	• Botulism • GI • Wound • Inhalation	• No antimicrobial recommended as they increase toxin load
	Clostridium tetani	R: Metronidazole A: Penicillin G erythromycin, tetracycline, clindamycin	• Usually follows contaminated wound	• Tetanus immune globulin • Rare in US
	Clostridium difficile	R: Metronidazole, vancomycin (oral only) A: Fidaxomicin	• Pseudomembraneous colitis	• Severe = PO vancomycin • Mild to moderate = metronidazole
	Clostridium perfringens	R: Penicillin G +/– clindamycin A: Doxycycline May also use piperacillin/tazobactam, cefazolin, cefoxitin, carbapenems	• Food poisoning; self-limiting • Gas gangrene	• Clindamycin in combination therapy; surgical intervention often required

(continued)

Organism Type	Specific Organisms	Recommended (R) and Alternative (A) Treatment	Common Types of Related Infections	Comments
Anaerobic gram negative rods (bacilli)	*Bacteroides fragilis*	R: Metronidazole A: Cefoxitin, carbapenems, pipera-cillin/tazobactam, ampicillin/sulbactam, cefotetan, amoxicillin/clavulanate, tigecycline, moxifloxacin (if susceptible)	• Intra-abdominal • PID • SSTIs	• Difficult to identify in lab • Increasing resistance • Susceptibilities should guide therapy
Anaerobic gram positive cocci	*Peptococcus* and *peptostreptococcus*	Sensitive to many antimicrobials R: Penicillin, amoxicillin, clindamycin, imipenem/cilastatin, β-lactam/β-lactamase combinations A: Vancomycin, moxifloxacin, levofloxacin, linezolid, daptomycin	• Aspiration PNA • Bacteremia • Dental infections • Endocarditis • Female GU infections • Intra-abdominal • SSTIs	• Oral/GI anaerobes • Oftentimes involved in poly-microbial infections
Atypical	*Chlamydophila pneumoniae*	R: Doxycycline A: FQ or macrolides	• Pneumonia	• Common in young adults • Also known as "walking pneumonia"
	Mycoplasma pneumoniae	R: Doxycycline A: FQ or macrolides		
	Legionella pneumophila	R: Levofloxacin, moxifloxacin A: Azithromycin		• Water is a typical reservoir • Older patients at risk

I.3 DOES THE PATIENT HAVE ANY HEALTHCARE-ASSOCIATED RISK FACTORS?

EVALUATING HEALTHCARE-ASSOCIATED RISK FACTORS

It is important to evaluate patients for all potential healthcare-associated risk factors as this ultimately affects the targeted pathogens and subsequent antimicrobial therapy selection. Patients may fall into any of the following risk categories for infections with multidrug-resistant organisms:

Low risk—Patients from the community setting with none of the risk factors below.

Mild risk—Patients who have any of the following risk factors:
- Hospitalization for ≥48 hours within 90 days
- Current hospitalization >5 days
- Residence in a nursing home or extended-care facility
- Antimicrobial use within 90 days
- Home infusion therapy (e.g., antimicrobials, chemotherapy, etc.) or home wound care
- Chronic dialysis within 30 days
- Family member in same residence with multidrug-resistant pathogens

High risk—Patients who have any of the following risk factors:
- Broad spectrum antimicrobial therapy in the last 90 days
  ○ Consider spectrum of activity, multiple courses, etc.
- Residence in a nursing home or extended-care facility plus other risk factors on this list
- Chronically ventilated patients
- Colonization or repeated infection with multidrug-resistant pathogens
- Chronic steroid or therapy with immunomodulators (TNF-alpha inhibitors, monoclonal antibodies, etc.)

Some patients may fall into more than one risk category. It is important to consider the type and level of risk when selecting antimicrobial therapy. For example, consider the following scenarios:

Case 1: A 54-yo-male presents to the emergency department with a large erythematous, purulent carbuncle on his left buttock. He has hypertension that is controlled with lisinopril and hydrochlorothiazide. This is his first skin and soft tissue infection, has no recent hospitalizations or antimicrobial exposure.

> **Risk Explanation:** This case represents a patient with no risk factors for multidrug-resistant organisms.

Case 2: A 34-yo-female presents to the hospital with shortness of breath, fever, increased respiratory rate, and productive cough. She has a past medical history of allergy-induced asthma and was treated 2.5 months ago with a 5-day course of cephalexin for uncomplicated cystitis. Her current chest X-ray reveals a left lower lobe infiltrate and is diagnosed with community-acquired pneumonia.

Risk Explanation: This case describes a patient who had a course of a narrow spectrum antimicrobial for an unrelated infection just shy of the 90-day risk factor cut-off. She may be at mild risk for some resistance; however, she should still receive appropriate therapy for community-acquired pneumonia targeting the most common organisms such as *S. pneumoniae*, *H. influenzae*, and atypical organisms with a respiratory fluoroquinolone or ceftriaxone plus azithromycin, etc.

Case 3: A 72-yo-male is transferred from a local long-term care facility to the emergency department with increased agitation, hypotension, fever, and leukocytosis. He had a stroke one year ago and has a history of repeated hospital admissions for infections. His last admission was three weeks ago for a urinary tract infection with subsequent bacteremia caused by *Enterobacter aerogenes* for which he just completed a 14-day course of meropenem. Since his stroke, he is in a chronic vegetative state, chronically ventilated, and is receiving enteral nutrition via PEG tube. His urinalysis is markedly abnormal, and urine and blood cultures are pending.

Risk Explanation: This case involves a high-risk patient with multiple risk factors, and empiric therapy should be broad enough to encompass the high likelihood of multidrug-resistant organisms.

PART II

What Is the Suspected Source of Infection and What Organisms Are Typically Associated with Infection at This Site?

II.1 BACTERIAL MENINGITIS

Bacterial Meningitis		Comments
Definition	**Bacterial meningitis:** bacterial infection of the meninges **Fungal meningitis:** fungal infection of the meninges **Viral meningitis:** viral infection of the meninges	Meninges are the protective membranes of the brain and spinal cord.
CSF Analysis	**Cerebrospinal fluid (CSF) in a noninfected patient is typically:** • Clear and sterile • Protein <50 mg/dL • CSF glucose is approximately 50–66% of serum glucose • pH = 7.4 • WBC <5 cells/mm³ (100% lymphocytes)	

Type	Normal	Bacterial	Viral
WBC (cells/mm³)	<5	1,000–5,000	100–1,000
Differential	Monocytes	PMN	Lymphocytes
Protein (mg/dL)	<50	100–500	30–150
Glucose (mg/dL)	50–66% serum value	<40 (60% serum)	<30–70

Common Offending Pathogens		
Gram +: • Group B streptococcus • *Listeria monocytogenes* • *Streptococcus pneumoniae* • *Nocardia*		
Gram −: • *Haemophilus influenzae* • *Neisseria meningitidis*		
Atypical: • Mycobacterium tuberculosis		
Viruses: • Arbovirus • Enteroviruses (Echovirus, Coxsackie viruses type A and B) • Herpes simplex virus • Human immunodeficiency virus (HIV) • Lymphocytic choriomeningitis virus • Mumps		

Bacterial Meningitis		Comments
Common Offending Pathogens	**Fungi:** **Most common** • *Coccidioides immitis* • *Cryptococcus neoformans* • *Histoplasma capsulatum* **Less common** • *Aspergillus* spp. • *Blastomyces dermatitidis* • *Candida* spp. • *Sporothrix schenckii*	
	Presumed bacterial pathogen differs based on age and other predisposing factors:	

Age	Bacterial Pathogens
<1 mo	• *Escherichia coli* • *Listeria monocytogenes* • *Streptococcus agalactiae*
1–23 mo	• *Escherichia coli* • *Haemophilus influenzae* • *Neisseria meningitidis* • *Streptococcus agalactiae* • *Streptococcus pneumoniae*
2–50 yr	• *Neisseria meningitidis* • *Streptococcus pneumoniae*
>50 yr	• Aerobic gram-negative bacilli • *Listeria monocytogenes* • *Neisseria meningitidis* • *Streptococcus pneumoniae*

Predisposing Factor	Bacterial Pathogens
Basilar skull fracture	• Group B streptococci • *Haemophilus influenza* • *Streptococcus pneumoniae*
Penetrating head trauma or post neurosurgery	• Coagulase-negative staphylococci • *Pseudomonas aeruginosa* • *Staphylococcus aureus*
Infected CSF shunt	• Coagulase-negative staphylococci • *Propionibacterium acnes* • *Pseudomonas aeruginosa* • *Staphylococcus aureus*

Bacterial Meningitis	Comments

Empiric Treatment of Choice
 	
	Age / **Empiric Therapy**
	
	 <1 mo — • Ampicillin plus cefotaxime • Ampicillin plus aminoglycoside
	
	 1–23 mo — Vancomycin plus a third-generation cephalosporin (ceftriaxone or cefotaxime)
	
	 2–50 yr — Vancomycin plus a third-generation cephalosporin (ceftriaxone or cefotaxime)
	
	 >50 yr — Vancomycin plus ampicillin plus a third-generation cephalosporin (ceftriaxone or cefotaxime)
	
	 Predisposing Factor / **Empiric Therapy**
	
	 Basilar skull fracture — Vancomycin plus a third-generation cephalosporin (ceftriaxone or cefotaxime)
	
	 Penetrating head trauma — • Vancomycin plus cefepime • Vancomycin plus ceftazidime • Vancomycin plus meropenem
	
	 Postneurosurgery — • Vancomycin plus cefepime • Vancomycin plus ceftazidime • Vancomycin plus meropenem
	
	 CSF shunt — • Vancomycin plus cefepime • Vancomycin plus ceftazidime • Vancomycin plus meropenem
		• Antimicrobial therapy should be started as soon as possible
		 • Bactericidal antimicrobials preferred over bacteriostatic antimicrobials
		 • Dual β-lactam treatment is rarely indicated
		 • Ceftriaxone plus ampicillin is acceptable for empiric therapy for the young and old to cover Streptococcus and Listeria
		 • Role of dexamethasone is controversial:
		  ○ **Pro:** said to reduce inflammation, which will prevent further neurological sequelae
		  ○ **Con:** reducing inflammation can also decrease antibiotic penetration
		  ○ **Children**
		   • Studies have shown improved outcomes with *H. influenzae* type B meningitis
		  ○ **Adults**
		   • Studies have shown some improved outcomes with pneumococcal meningitis

Bacterial Meningitis		Comments
Alternative Empiric Treatment Options	**Presumed Pathogen** / **Therapy**	

	Presumed Pathogen	Therapy
Alternative Empiric Treatment Options	*Escherichia coli* and other Enterobacteriaceae	Cefepime, meropenem, aztreonam, moxifloxacin, TMP-SMX
	Haemophilus influenzae	Chloramphenicol, cefepime, meropenem, moxifloxacin
	Listeria monocytogenes	TMP-SMX, meropenem
	Neisseria meningitidis	Penicillin G, ampicillin, chloramphenicol, moxifloxacin, aztreonam
	Pseudomonas aeruginosa	Aztreonam, ciprofloxacin, meropenem
	Staphylococcus aureus	TMP-SMX, linezolid
	Streptococcus agalactiae	Ceftriaxone, cefotaxime
	Streptococcus pneumoniae	Meropenem, moxifloxacin

	Pathogen Isolated		Comments
	Pathogen	**Therapy**	
Definitive Therapy	*Streptococcus pneumoniae*	Vancomycin plus a third-generation cephalosporin (ceftriaxone or cefotaxime)	• For CSF shunt infections/ventriculitis, intraventricular antimicrobial therapy should be considered.
	Neisseria meningitidis	Third-generation cephalosporin (ceftriaxone or cefotaxime)	
	Listeria monocytogenes	Ampicillin or penicillin G (consider adding an aminoglycoside)	
	Streptococcus agalactiae	Ampicillin or penicillin G (consider adding an aminoglycoside)	
	Haemophilus influenzae	Third-generation cephalosporin (ceftriaxone or cefotaxime)	
	Escherichia coli and other Enterobacteriaceae	Third-generation cephalosporin (ceftriaxone or cefotaxime)	
	Pseudomonas aeruginosa	• Cefepime • Ceftazidime	
	Staphylococcus aureus	• Nafcillin or Oxacillin (MSSA) • Vancomycin (MRSA)	

Bacterial Meningitis			Comments
Definitive Therapy	**Pathogen Isolated**		
	Pathogen	**Therapy**	
	Enterococcus	• Ampicillin plus gentamicin (ampicillin sensitive) • Vancomycin plus gentamicin (ampicillin resistant) • Linezolid (ampicillin and vancomycin resistant)	
	Recommended Antimicrobial Doses for Intraventricular Administration		
	Antimicrobial	**Daily Intraventricular Dose**	
	Amikacin	5–50 mg (average 30 mg)	
	Colistin	10 mg	
	Gentamicin	4–8 mg adults 1–2 mg pediatrics	
	Polymyxin B	5 mg adults 2 mg pediatrics	
	Quinupristin/dalfopristin	2–5 mg	
	Tobramycin	5–20 mg	
	Vancomycin	10–20 mg	
Penetration of Drug into the CSF	Therapeutic levels without inflammation	Isoniazid, metronidazole, rifampin, sulfonamides, TMP	Important to determine penetration of drug into the CSF
	Therapeutic levels with inflammation	Acyclovir, aztreonam, ceftazidime, ceftriaxone, ciprofloxacin, fluconazole, foscarnet, flucytosine, ganciclovir, linezolid, penicillins, vancomycin	
	Nontherapeutic levels regardless of inflammation	First- and second-generation cephalosporins, aminoglycosides, amphotericin B, clindamycin, itraconazole, ketoconazole	

	Bacterial Meningitis		Comments
Duration of Therapy	**Microorganism**	**Duration of Therapy, Days**	Duration of therapy depends on identified pathogen and clinical status If concomitant bacteremia, treatment should be at least 14 days
	Neisseria meningitidis	7	
	Haemophilus influenzae	7	
	Streptococcus pneumoniae	10–14	
	Streptococcus agalactiae	14–21	
	Aerobic gram-negative bacilli	21	
	Listeria monocytogenes	≥21	

REFERENCES

Nau R, Sörgel F, Eiffert H. Penetration of drugs through the blood-cerebrospinal fluid/blood-brain-barrier for treatment of central nervous system infections. *Clin Microbiol Rev.* 2010 Oct;23(4):858–883.

Tunkel AR, Hartman BJ, Kaplan SL, et al. Practice guidelines for the management of bacterial meningitis. *Clin Infect Dis.* 2004;39:1267–1284.

II.2   CANDIDIASIS

	Candidiasis	Comments
Definitions	**Candidiasis:** Fungal infection caused by *Candida* spp.	**Risk factors:** • Broad-spectrum antimicrobial use • Central venous catheters • Immunosuppressive agents • Implantable prosthetic devices • Multiple anatomic sites with colonization • Neutropenia • Chronic parenteral nutrition • Renal replacement therapy in ICU patients • Burn patients
Offending Pathogens	*Candida albicans* *Candida glabrata* *Candida krusei* *Candida lusitaniae* *Candida parapsilosis* *Candida tropicalis*	*Candida parapsilosis* may be resistant to echinocandins *Candida glabrata* may be susceptible dose dependent to azoles and resistant to amphotericin B (AmB) *Candida krusei* is resistant to fluconazole and flucytosine and may be resistant to itraconazole and AmB *Candida lusitaniae* may be resistant to AmB

	Candidiasis	Comments
Empiric Therapy for Suspected Candidiasis	**Non-neutropenic adults** *Preferred* • Echinocandin • Fluconazole 800 mg (12 mg/kg) load, then 400 mg (6 mg/kg) daily *Alternative* Lipid formulation of Amphotericin (LAmB) 3–5 mg/kg/day or Conventional Amphotericin B (AmB-d) 0.5–1 mg/kg/day	**Echinocandins**: anidulafungin, caspofungin, and micafungin Start with an echinocandin for severe infections, in patients who have had recent exposure to azoles, or if high local prevalence of fluconazole-resistant strains Duration is dependent on confirmed diagnosis and severity and site of infection
	Neutropenic adults *Preferred* LAmB 3–5 mg/kg/day or echinocandin or voriconazole 400 mg (6 mg/kg) Q12h × 2 doses then 200 mg (3 mg/kg) Q12h *Alternative* Fluconazole 800 mg (12 mg/kg) load, then 400 mg (6 mg/kg) daily or itraconazole 200 mg (3 mg/kg) Q12h	In a patient with an unidentified source and persistent fever despite antimicrobial therapy after 4 days, initiate antifungal therapy Avoid azoles empirically in patients who received azole prophylaxis
Candidemia Initial Treatment	**Non-neutropenic adults** *Preferred* Fluconazole 800 mg (12 mg/kg) load, then 400 mg (6 mg/kg) daily or an echinocandin *Alternative* LAmB 3–5 mg/kg/day or AmB-d 0.5–1 mg/kg/day or voriconazole 400 mg (6 mg/kg) Q12h × 2 doses then 200 mg (3 mg/kg) Q12h	Consider echinocandin for severe illness or patients with recent azole use May de-escalate to fluconazole once cultures are finalized if susceptible Remove intravascular catheters if possible Duration of therapy should be 14 days after first negative blood culture and resolution of signs and symptoms Ophthalmological exam recommended for all patients
	Neutropenic adults *Preferred* Echinocandin or LAmB 3–5 mg/kg/day	Echinocandin or LAmB preferred for most patients Fluconazole may be considered for patients who are not critically ill and have not had recent azole exposure

	Candidiasis	Comments
Candidemia Initial Treatment	*Alternative* Fluconazole 800 mg (12 mg/kg) load, then 400 mg (6 mg/kg) daily or voriconazole 400 mg (6 mg/kg) Q12h × 2 doses then 200 mg (3 mg/kg) Q12h	Voriconazole should be considered when additional mold (e.g., *Aspergillus* spp.) coverage is needed Source control is an essential component to management, including line removal, when possible
CNS Candidiasis	*Preferred* LAmB 3–5 mg/kg/day +/– flucytosine 25 mg/kg Q6h × several weeks, then fluconazole 400–800 mg (6–12 mg/kg) day *Alternative* For patients who cannot tolerate LAmB, fluconazole 400–800 mg (6–12 mg/kg) day	Treat until all signs and symptoms have resolved Source control is an essential component to management, including line removal, when possible
Candida Endophthalmitis	*Preferred* AmB-d 0.7–1 mg/kg + flucytosine 25 mg/kg Q6h or fluconazole 6–12 mg/kg/day Surgical intervention is oftentimes required *Alternative* LAmB 3–5 mg/kg/day or voriconazole 6 mg/kg Q12h × 2 doses then 3–4 mg/kg Q12h or echinocandin	Treatment duration is at least 4–6 weeks Examinations should be repeated to confirm resolution Intravitreal administration may be required
Mucocutaneous Candidiasis	**Oropharyngeal** *Preferred* Clotrimazole troches 10 mg 5 times/day, or nystatin suspension or pastilles Q6h, or fluconazole 100–200 mg day *Alternative* Itraconazole oral solution 200 mg daily or posaconazole 400 mg daily or voriconazole 200 mg Q12h or echinocandin or AmB-d 0.3 mg/kg/day	Mild disease: clotrimazole or nystatin Moderate-to-severe disease: fluconazole Treat for 7–14 days Consider alternative agents for refractory disease
	Esophageal *Preferred* Fluconazole 200–400 mg (3–6 mg/kg) daily or echinocandin or AmB-d 0.3–0.7 mg/kg/day	Oral fluconazole preferred Treat for 14–21 days AmB-d or echinocandin may be used for refractory disease

	Candidiasis	Comments
Mucocutaneous Candidiasis	*Alternative* Itraconazole oral solution 200 mg daily or posaconazole 400 mg PO Q12h or voriconazole 200 mg Q12h	
	Vulvovaginal Topical agents or fluconazole 150 mg × 1 dose	Repeat doses of fluconazole 150 mg once weekly may be considered for recurrent disease
Lower Respiratory Candidiasis	Treatment not recommended	Rare for Candida to cause true lower respiratory tract infection; Candida isolated in the lower respiratory track typically considered colonization
Urinary Tract Candidiasis	**Asymptomatic cystitis** Treatment not indicated unless patients at high risk or undergoing urologic procedures High risk: Fluconazole 400 mg (6 mg/kg) daily if patient stable LAmB 3–5 mg/kg/day or AmB-d 0.5–0.7 mg/kg/day for severely ill patients (change to fluconazole once stable) Undergoing urologic procedure: Fluconazole 200–400 mg (3–6 mg/kg) daily or AmB-d 0.3–0.6 mg/kg/day for several days pre- and post-procedure	High risk: neonates and neutropenic adults
	Symptomatic cystitis *Preferred* Fluconazole 200 mg (3 mg/kg) daily for 14 days *Alternative* AmB-d 0.3–0.6 mg/kg/day for 1–7 days or flucytosine 25 mg/kg Q6h for 7–10 days	Consider alternative therapy for fluconazole-resistant organisms AmB-d bladder irrigation may also be considered for refractory fluconazole-resistant organisms
	Pyelonephritis *Preferred* Fluconazole 200–400 mg (3–6 mg/kg) daily for 14 days	Fungal pyelonephritis is rare

	Candidiasis	Comments
Urinary Tract Candidiasis	*Alternative* AmB-d 0.5–0.7 mg/kg/day +/– flucytosine 25 mg/kg Q6h or flucytosine 25 mg/kg Q6h alone for 14 days	
	Fungal balls Surgical removal and Fluconazole 200–400 mg (3–6 mg/kg) daily or AmB-d 0.5–0.7 mg/kg/day +/– flucytosine 25 mg/kg Q6h	Local AmB-d irrigation may also be considered
Candida Osteomyelitis	*Preferred* Fluconazole 400 mg (6 mg/ kg) daily for 6–12 months or LAmB 3–5 mg/kg/day for several weeks, then fluco- nazole for 6–12 weeks	Treat for 6–12 months Surgical intervention is oftentimes necessary
	Alternative Echinocandin or AmB-d 0.5–1 mg/kg/day for several weeks then fluconazole for 6–12 months	
Candida Endocarditis	*Preferred* LAmB 3–5 mg/kg +/– flucyto- sine 25 mg/kg Q6h or AmB-d 0.6–1 mg/kg/day +/– flucytosine 25 mg/kg Q6h or echinocandin	Valve replacement strongly recommended Fluconazole 400–800 mg (6–12 mg/kg) as chronic suppression is recommended for patients who are unable to undergo surgical intervention High rates of mortality
	Alternative De-escalate therapy to fluco- nazole 400–800 mg (6–12 mg/ kg) daily for a patient with a susceptible organism with negative blood cultures	
Chronic Disseminated Candidiasis	*Preferred* Fluconazole 400 mg (6 mg/kg) daily if patient stable LAmB 3–5 mg/kg/day or AmB-d 0.5–0.7 mg/kg/day for severely ill patients (change to fluco- nazole once stable)	Transition from LAmB or AmB-d to fluconazole is preferred after several weeks in stable patients Treatment should be continued until resolution (several months) or through periods of immunosuppression
	Alternative Echinocandin for several weeks followed by fluconazole	

II.3   CATHETER-RELATED BLOODSTREAM INFECTIONS

Catheter-Related Bloodstream Infections (CRBSI)		Comments
Definition	**Catheter-related bloodstream infection:** infection caused by catheters that become colonized with bacteria, which subsequently seed the bloodstream **Central venous catheter (CVC):** a catheter that is passed through a large vein; commonly referred to as a central line **Peripherally inserted central venous catheter (PICC):** catheters inserted into a peripheral vein and advanced toward the heart through increasingly larger veins	
Clinical Presentation	• Fever • Erythema • Inflammation or purulence at the insertion site • Pain • Hemodynamic instability • Altered mental status • Catheter dysfunction	
Common Offending Pathogens	**Gram +:** Coagulase negative *Staphylococcus, Staphylococcus aureus, Enterococcus faecalis/faecium* **Gram –:** *P. aeruginosa, E. coli, K. pneumoniae, Enterobacter* spp., *Serratia marscescens, Acinetobacter* spp., *Burkholderia cepacia* **Fungal:** *Candida* spp.	
Empiric Therapy	Vancomycin for CRBSI in healthcare settings Add gram-negative coverage (including *Pseudomonas*) for neutropenic or septic patients (i.e., cefepime, piperacillin/tazobactam, carbapenem)	Need coverage for MRSA and MRSE • Alternative to vancomycin (i.e., daptomycin) • Organism and susceptibilities will guide therapy

Treatment of Choice	Pathogen	Drug	Dose	Comment	In general, systemic antimicrobial therapy is **NOT** required in the following circumstances: • Positive catheter tip culture with no clinical signs of infection
	Gram (+) cocci				
	MSSA	Nafcillin or oxacillin	2 g IV Q4h	Cefazolin or vancomycin if PCN allergic	
	MRSA	Vancomycin	15 mg/kg IV Q12h	May use daptomycin or ceftazidime if vancomycin resistant	

Catheter-Related Bloodstream Infections (CRBSI)				Comments
Treatment of Choice				• Positive blood cultures from catheter with negative cultures through peripheral vein • Phlebitis with no infection • Type of pathogen is important for guiding treatment decisions • Catheters should be removed if due to *S. aureus*, *P. aeruginosa*, fungi, or mycobacteria • Antibiotic lock therapy may be used in patients whose catheters cannot be removed

Pathogen	Drug	Dose	Comment
Coagulase-negative staphylococci			
MSSE	Nafcillin or oxacillin	2 g IV Q4h	Cefazolin or vancomycin if PCN allergic
MRSE	Vancomycin	15 mg/kg IV Q12h	May use daptomycin or linezolid if vancomycin resistant

Pathogen	Drug	Dose	Comment
Enterococcus faecalis/Enterococcus faecium			
Ampicillin susceptible	• Ampicillin ± • Gentamicin	• 2 g IV Q4h • 1 mg/kg IV Q8h	Avoid quinupristin/ dalfopristin if *E. faecalis*
Ampicillin resistant, vancomycin susceptible	• Vancomycin ± • Gentamicin	• 15 mg/kg IV Q12h • 1 mg/kg IV Q8h	
Ampicillin resistant, vancomycin resistant	• Linezolid or • Daptomycin	• 600 mg Q12h • 6 mg/kg IV daily	

Gram-negative bacilli			
Pathogen	Drug	Dose	Comment
***Escherichia coli* and *Klebsiella* species**			
ESBL negative	Ceftriaxone	1–2 g IV daily	Ciprofloxacin or aztreonam may be used
ESBL positive	• Ertapenem or • Imipenem/ Cilastatin or • Meropenem or • Doripenem	• 1 g IV daily • 500 mg IV Q6h • 1 g IV Q8h • 500 mg IV Q8h	Ciprofloxacin or aztreonam may be used

Catheter-Related Bloodstream Infections (CRBSI)			
Treatment of Choice	**Gram-negative bacilli**		
	Pathogen	**Drug**	**Dose**	**Comment**
	Enterobacter species and *Serratia marcescens*	• Ertapenem or • Imipenem/ Cilastatin or • Meropenem	• 1 g IV daily • 500 mg IV Q6h • 1 g IV Q8h	Cefepime or ciprofloxacin may be used
	Acinetobacter species	• Ampicillin/ sulbactam or • Imipenem/ Cilastatin or • Meropenem	• 3 g IV Q6h • 500 mg IV Q6h • 1 g IV Q8h	
	Stenotro-phomonas maltophilia	TMP/SMX	3–5 mg/kg IV Q8h Dose based on TMP compo-nent	Ticarcillin/clavulanate may be used
	Pseudomonas aeruginosa	• Cefepime or • Imipenem/ Cilastatin or • Meropenem or • Piperacillin/ tazobactam ± • Amikacin or • Tobramycin	• 2 g IV Q8h • 500 mg IV Q6h • 1 g IV Q8h • 4.5 g IV Q6h • 15 mg/kg IV Q24h • 5–7 mg/kg IV Q24h	Typically see this patho-gen in patients who are: • Neutropenic • Septic • Colonized previously with *Pseudomonas* • May consider fluoro-quinolones if suscep-tible

Catheter-Related Bloodstream Infections (CRBSI)			
Treatment of Choice	*Burkholderia cepacia*	• TMP/SMX or • Imipenem/ Cilastatin or • Meropenem	• 3–5 mg/kg IV Q8h • 500 mg IV Q6h • 1 g IV Q8h	

Fungi			
Pathogen	**Drug**	**Dose**	**Comment**
Candida albicans or other *Candida* species	• Caspofungin or • Micafungin or • Fluconazole	• 70 mg IV LD then 50 mg IV daily • 100 mg IV daily • 400–600 mg daily	Risk factors for fungal CRBSI: • Patients receiving TPN • Prolonged use of broad-spectrum antibiotics • Hematologic malignancy • Bone marrow or solid organ transplant recipients • Femoral catheterization • Fluconazole should be avoided in *C. Krusei* CRBSI
Ochrobacterium	• TMP/SMX or • Ciprofloxacin	• 3–5 mg/kg IV Q8h • 400 mg IV Q12h	
Malassezia furfur	Amphotericin B	AmBisome: • 3–5 mg/kg IV daily Abelcet: • 5 mg/kg IV daily	

Catheter-Related Bloodstream Infections (CRBSI)		Comments
Duration of Therapy	• Uncomplicated CRBSI with negative blood cultures following catheter removal: 10 to 14 days • Prosthetic valve: 4–6 weeks • Persistent bacteremia >72 hours despite catheter removal: 4–6 weeks	Day one of anti-infective therapy is the first day when negative blood cultures are obtained
Antibiotic Lock Therapy	<table><tr><td>**Antibiotic and Dosage**</td><td>**Heparin or Saline (units/mL)**</td><td>**Dwell Time**</td></tr><tr><td>Cefazolin 5 mg/mL</td><td>2,500 or 5,000</td><td>48 hours</td></tr><tr><td>Vancomycin 5 mg/mL</td><td>2,500 or 5,000</td><td>48 hours</td></tr><tr><td>Ceftazidime 10 mg/mL</td><td>100</td><td>48 hours</td></tr><tr><td>Gentamicin 1 mg/mL</td><td>2,500</td><td>48 hours</td></tr><tr><td>Cefazolin 10 mg/mL and gentamicin 5 mg/mL</td><td>5,000</td><td>48 hours</td></tr><tr><td>Vancomycin 10 mg/mL and gentamicin 5 mg/mL</td><td>5,000</td><td>48 hours</td></tr></table>	Use antibiotic lock therapy if trying to salvage the catheter Not to be used as mono-therapy; use in conjunction with systemic anti-microbials Typical duration of antibiotic lock therapy is 14 days. Antifungal or ethanol locks may also be utilized
Prevention of CRBSI	**Catheter site care:** May disinfect skin prior to catheter insertion and during dressing changes with 2% chlorhexidine-based preparation. (May also use tincture of iodine or 70% alcohol.) **Catheter site dressing regimens:** Topical antibiotic ointments or creams should NOT be used on insertion sites (except dialysis catheters).	

REFERENCES

Mermel LA, Allon M, Bouza E, et al. Clinical practice guidelines for the diagnosis and management of intravascular catheter-related infection: 2009 update by the Infectious Diseases Society of America. *Clin Infect Dis.* 2009;49:1–45.

O'Grady NP, Alexander M, Burns LA, et al. Guidelines for the prevention of intravascular catheter-related infections. *Clin Infect Dis.* 2011:52(1May):e1–e32.

Vercaigne LM, Zelenitsky SA, Findlay I, et al. An in vitro evaluation of the antibiotic/heparin lock to sterilize central venous haemodialysis catheters. *J Antimicrob Chemother.* 2002;49:693.

II.4 *CLOSTRIDIUM DIFFICILE* INFECTION

	Clostridium difficile Infection (CDI)	Comments
Definitions	*Clostridium difficile* **Infection (CDI):** infection of the colon that causes an expansive spectrum of disease (from asymptomatic colonization to fulminant pseudomembraneous colitis) and is based on the following criteria: • Presence of symptoms (diarrhea: ≥3 loose or watery stools over 24 hours for 2 consecutive days) • Ileus • Positive stool test detecting the presence of *C. difficile* or its toxins • Presence of pseudomembranes on endoscopy • Positive PCR in a patient without symptoms indicates colonization	**Risk factors:** • Age >64 years • Duration of hospital stay • Gastrointestinal surgery • HIV infection • Receipt of chemotherapeutic agents • Recent antimicrobial use **Complications:** • Colectomy • Death • Dehydration • Electrolyte abnormalities • Hypotension • Ileus • Renal failure • Sepsis • Toxic megacolon High recurrence rates (15–35%); rate increases with each recurrence

Testing	**Test**	**Advantages**	**Limitations**	Stool testing should be performed *only* on unformed stool from symptomatic patients (3 liquid stools within 24 hours without an identifiable cause) Should not use as test of cure as assays may remain positive for weeks
	Stool culture	Very sensitive	Most often associated with false-positive results*; labor-intensive; requires 48–96 hours for results	
	Antigen detection	Rapid tests (<1 hour)	Must be combined with toxin testing to verify diagnosis	
	Enzyme immunoassay	Same-day test; detects toxin A, or A and B	Less sensitive than tissue culture cytotoxicity assay	

*Nontoxigenic *C. difficile* strains test positive

Clostridium difficile Infection (CDI)			Comments
Testing			

Test	Advantages	Limitations
Tissue culture	More sensitive than enzyme immunoassay	Detects toxin B only; costly; requires 24–48 hours for a final result
PCR	Sensitivity >94% and specificity >95%	Detects asymptomatic colonization

Prevention	• Appropriate antimicrobial stewardship • Hand hygiene compliance • Patient isolation with contact precautions while hospitalized • Environmental cleaning	Hand hygiene should include soap and water; alcohol-based hand sanitizers do not kill spores
Offending Pathogen	*Clostridium difficile*	Anaerobic spore-forming gram-positive bacillus Produces toxin A (enterotoxin) and toxin B (cytotoxin)
Initial Episode, Mild or Moderate Treatment • WBC <15,000 cells/μL and • SCr <1.5 times premorbid level	Metronidazole 500 mg PO Q8h May give metronidazole IV if not taking PO Use of metronidazole beyond 14 days is discouraged due to the risk of adverse effects (neuropathy)	Discontinue offending antimicrobial or de-escalate antimicrobial therapy when possible Correct fluid losses/electrolyte imbalances and avoid antimotility agents (including opioids), due to the risk of toxic megacolon
Initial Episode, Severe Treatment • WBC ≥15,000 cells/μL or • SCr ≥1.5 times premorbid level	Vancomycin 125 mg PO Q6h	May prepare oral vancomycin suspension from IV formulation Rifaximin is a nonabsorbed rifamycin antibiotic that has shown promise in patients with multiple CDI recurrences; 400–800 mg PO in 2 or 3 divided doses (200 mg 2–3 times daily or 400 mg twice daily) for 2 weeks **after** completion of traditional therapy

Clostridium difficile Infection (CDI)		Comments
Initial Episode Severe, Complicated Treatment • Hypotension • Shock • Ileus • Megacolon	Vancomycin 500 mg PO Q6h or NG tube plus metronidazole 500 mg IV Q8h If complete ileus, consider adding rectal instillation of vancomycin	Fidaxomicin 200 mg PO Q12h for 10 days is an alternative; however, very costly (10-day course ~$2,400) Other emerging therapies include nitazoxanide, IVIG, monoclonal antibodies, and fecal transplant Bile acid sequestrants (e.g., cholestyramine, colestipol) are **NOT recommended** for use in the management of CDI as they commonly cause abdominal distension and may bind oral vancomycin Therapy with microorganisms (probiotics) are **NOT recommended** and should be avoided due to the risk of microbial translocation
First Recurrence Treatment	Same as for initial episode	
Second Recurrence Treatment	Vancomycin tapered, pulsed regimen: Weeks 1–2: 125 mg PO Q6h Week 3: 125 mg PO Q12h Week 4: 125 mg PO daily Week 5: 125 mg PO every other day Week 6: 125 mg PO every 3rd day	
Duration of Therapy	10–14 days	

REFERENCES

Cohen SH, Gerding DN, Johnson S, et al. Clinical practice guidelines for *Clostridium difficile* infection in adults: 2010 update by the Society for Healthcare Epidemiology of America (SHEA) and the Infectious Diseases Society of America (IDSA). *Infect Control Hosp Epidemiol.* 2010;31:431–455.

Surawicz CM, Brandt LJ, Binion DG, et al. Guidelines for diagnosis, treatment, and prevention of *Clostridium difficile* infections. *Am J Gastroenterol.* 2013;108:478–498.

❖   ❖   ❖

II.5   INFECTIVE ENDOCARDITIS

Infective Endocarditis		Comments
Definition	**Endocarditis**: inflammation of the lining of the heart valves and chambers. **Infective endocarditis (IE):** infection of the lining of the heart valves and chambers.	• Definition of IE based on modified Duke criteria
Modified Duke Criteria	DEFINITIVE IE **Pathological criteria** • (+) cultured microorganisms or evidence of vegetation; or pathological lesions; or intracardiac abscess showing active endocarditis **Clinical criteria** • 2 major criteria; or • 1 major criterion and 3 minor criteria; or • 5 minor criteria POSSIBLE IE • 1 major criterion and 1 minor criterion; or • 3 minor criteria	

Major Criteria	Minor Criteria
• Blood culture (+) for IE: at least 2 separate blood cultures for a typical IE organism: viridans streptococci, *S. bovis*, HACEK group, *S. aureus*, or *Enterococcus* spp. • Persistent bacteremia with any microorganism defined as: 2 (+) blood cultures drawn at least 12 hours apart; or 3 out of 3 (+) blood cultures drawn at least 1 hour apart or a majority of ≥4 blood cultures drawn during any time period • Single (+) blood culture or serology for *Coxiella burnetii* • Evidence of endocardial involvement • Echocardiogram (+) for IE ○ TEE strongly recommended for patients with prosthetic valves and TTE recommended as first test in other patients	• Predisposing condition: previous heart condition or IV drug use • Fever >38°C (100.4°F) • Embolic evidence: arterial or pulmonary emboli, mycotic aneurysm, intracranial hemorrhage, conjunctival hemorrhage, Janeway lesions • Immunologic evidence: glomerulonephritis, Osler nodes, Roth spots, (+) rheumatoid factor • (+) blood cultures that do not meet a major criterion or serologic evidence of active IE

Common Offending Pathogens	Most common bacterial cause of infective endocarditis: streptococci, staphylococci, and enterococci **Gram +:** • Coagulase negative (*S. epidermidis. S. lugdunensis*) • Coagulase positive (*S. aureus*) • Enterococci (*E. faecalis* and *E. faecium*) • Other streptococci (*S. bovis*) • *Viridans streptococcus*	

Infective Endocarditis		Comments
Common Offending Pathogens	**Gram −:** • Bartonella species • Enterobacteriaceae (Salmonella species, *E. coli*, *Serratia marcescens*, *P. mirabilis*, Klebsiella species) • Enterobacteriaceae (Salmonella species, *E. coli*, *Serratia marcescens*, *P. mirabilis*, Klebsiella species) • HACEK (*H. parainfluenzae*, H. aphrophilus, *H. influenza*, *H. paraphrophilus*, *Actinobacillus actinomycetemcomitans*, *Cardiobacterium hominis*, *Eikenella corrodens*, *Kingella kingae*, *K. denitrificans*) • *Pseudomonas aeruginosa*	
	Fungi: • *Aspergillus* spp. • *Candida* spp.	Fungal IE is rare. If diagnosed, surgical replacement of infected valve is warranted.

INFECTIVE ENDOCARDITIS—CULTURE PENDING

Valve	Empiric Treatment	Comments
Native	• Ampicillin–sulbactam 3 g IV Q6h plus • Gentamicin 1 mg/kg IV Q8h or • Vancomycin 15 mg/kg IV Q12h	Adjust vancomycin dose to achieve target trough of 10–20 mcg/mL Target gentamicin peak: 3–4 mcg/mL Target gentamicin trough: <1 mcg/mL Can often just monitor gentamicin trough to ensure drug clearance Consider the most likely pathogen based on risk factors or initial gram stain
Prosthetic	• Vancomycin 15 mg/kg IV Q12h plus • Gentamicin 1 mg/kg IV Q8h plus • Rifampin 600 mg PO Q24h	
	• Linezolid 600 mg IV Q12h or • Daptomycin ≥8 mg/kg IV Q24h	May be used in patients intolerant to vancomycin

INFECTIVE ENDOCARDITIS—CULTURE POSITIVE

Organism	Valve	Definitive Treatment	Duration (weeks)	Comments
Enterococcus spp. (PCN susceptible)	Native	• Ampicillin 2 g IV Q4h or • PCN G 3 million/units IV Q4h plus • Gentamicin 1 mg/kg IV Q8h	4–6	Target gentamicin peak: 3–4 mcg/mL Target gentamicin trough: <1 mcg/mL Streptomycin may be an alternative for gentamicin resistant strains

Organism	Valve	Definitive Treatment	Duration (weeks)	Comments
Enterococcus spp. (PCN susceptible)	Native	• Ampicillin 2 g IV Q4h plus • Ceftriaxone 2 g IV Q12h	6	Typically used when aminoglycoside is not an option
	Prosthetic	• Ampicillin 2 g IV Q4h or • PCN G 3 million/units IV Q4h plus • Gentamicin 1 mg/kg IV Q8h	6	Target gentamicin peak: 3–4 mcg/mL Target gentamicin trough: <1 mcg/mL Streptomycin may be an alternative for gentamicin-resistant strains
		• Ampicillin 2 g IV Q4h plus • Ceftriaxone 2 g IV Q12h	6	Typically used when aminoglycoside is not an option
Enterococcus spp. (PCN resistant)	Native	• Vancomycin 15 mg/kg IV Q12h plus • Gentamicin 1 mg/kg/IV Q8h	6	Target gentamicin peak: 3–4 mcg/mL Target gentamicin trough: <1 mcg/mL
	Prosthetic	• Vancomycin 15 mg/kg IV Q12h plus • Gentamicin 1 mg/kg/IV Q8h	6	
Enterococcus spp. (PCN, Aminoglycoside, and Vancomycin resistant)	Native	• Linezolid 600 mg IV/PO Q12h or • Daptomycin 10–12 mg/kg IV Q24h	>6	
	Prosthetic	• Linezolid 600 mg IV/PO Q12h or • Daptomycin 10–12 mg/kg IV Q24h	>6	
Methicillin-Susceptible S. aureus (MSSA)	Native	• Nafcillin or oxacillin 2 g IV Q4–6h	6	
		• Cefazolin 2 g IV Q8h	6	
	Prosthetic	• Nafcillin or oxacillin 2 g IV Q4–6h plus • Rifampin 300 mg IV or PO TID plus • Gentamicin 1 mg/kg IV Q8h	≥6 2 (gentamicin)	Target gentamicin peak: 3–4 mcg/mL Target gentamicin trough: <1 mcg/mL
		• Cefazolin 2 g IV Q8h	6	
Methicillin-Resistant S. aureus (MRSA)	Native	• Vancomycin 15 mg/kg IV Q12h	6	Adjust dose to achieve target trough of 10–20 mcg/mL
		• Daptomycin ≥8 mg/kg IV Q24h	6	

Organism	Valve	Definitive Treatment	Duration (weeks)	Comments
Methicillin-Resistant *S. aureus* (MRSA)	Prosthetic	• Vancomycin 15 mg/kg IV Q12h plus • Rifampin 300 mg IV or PO TID plus • Gentamicin 1 mg/kg IV Q8h	≥6 2 (gentamicin)	Adjust vancomycin dose to achieve target trough of 10–20 mcg/mL Target gentamicin peak: 3–4 mcg/mL Target gentamicin trough: <1 mcg/mL
Viridian Group Streptococci (VGS) and *Streptococcus gallolyticus (bovis)* (PCN susceptible)	Native	• PCN G 3 million/units IV Q4h or • Ceftriaxone 2 g IV/IM Q24h	4	
		• PCN G 3 million/units IV Q4h or • Ceftriaxone 2 g IV/IM Q24h plus • Gentamicin 3 mg/kg IV Q24h	2	May be used in patients with uncomplicated IE and respond quickly to treatment Gentamicin 3 mg/kg as a single dose preferred for VGS
		• Vancomycin 15 mg/kg IV Q12h	4	Alternative for patients who cannot tolerate PCN or ceftriaxone
	Prosthetic	• PCN G 4 million/units IV Q4h or • Ceftriaxone 2 g IV/IM Q24h with or without • Gentamicin 3 mg/kg IV Q24h	6 2 (gentamicin)	May be used in patients with uncomplicated IE and respond quickly to treatment Gentamicin 3 mg/kg as a single dose preferred for VGS
		• Vancomycin 15 mg/kg IV Q12h	6	Alternative for patients who cannot tolerate PCN or ceftriaxone
Viridian Group Streptococci (VGS) and *Streptococcus gallolyticus (bovis)* (PCN resistant)	Native	• PCN G 4 million/units IV Q4h plus • Gentamicin 3 mg/kg IV Q24h	4 2 (gentamicin)	Gentamicin 3 mg/kg as a single dose preferred for VGS
		• Vancomycin 15 mg/kg IV Q12h	4	Alternative for patients who cannot tolerate PCN or ceftriaxone
	Prosthetic	• PCN G 4 million/units IV Q4h or • Ceftriaxone 2 g IV/IM Q24h with or without • Gentamicin 3 mg/kg IV Q24h	6	Gentamicin 3 mg/kg as a single dose preferred for VGS
		• Vancomycin 15 mg/kg IV Q12h	6	Alternative for patients who cannot tolerate PCN or ceftriaxone

Organism	Valve	Definitive Treatment	Duration (weeks)	Comments
HACEK	Native	• Ceftriaxone 2 g IV/IM Q24h or • Ampicillin 2 g IV Q4h or • Ciprofloxacin 500 mg PO Q12h or 400 mg IV Q12h	4	HACEK organisms typically resistant to ampicillin and penicillin Levofloxacin or moxifloxacin may be substituted for ciprofloxacin
	Prosthetic	• Ceftriaxone 2 g IV/IM Q24h or • Ampicillin 2 g IV Q4h or • Ciprofloxacin 500 mg PO Q12h or 400 mg IV Q12h	4	

REFERENCES

Baddour LM, Wilson WR, Bayer AS, et al. Infective endocarditis: diagnosis, antimicrobial therapy, and management of complications: a scientific statement for healthcare professionals from the American Heart Association: endorsed by the Infectious Diseases Society of America. *Circulation.* 2015;132:1–53.

Gould FK, Denning DW, Elliott TSJ, et al. Guidelines for the diagnosis and antibiotic treatment of endocarditis in adults: a report of the working party of the British Society of Antimicrobial Chemotherapy. *J Antimicrob Chemother.* 2012;67:269–289.

Li JS, Sexton DJ, Mick N, et al. Proposed modifications to the Duke criteria for the diagnosis of infective endocarditis. *Clin Infect Dis.* 2000;30:633–638.

The Task Force on the Prevention, Diagnosis, and Treatment of Infective Endocarditis of the European Society of Cardiology (ESC). Guidelines on the prevention, diagnosis, and treatment of infective endocarditis (new version 2009). *Eur Heart J.* 2009;30:2369–2413.

Veverka A, Crouch MA. Infective endocarditis. In: DiPiro JT, Talbert RL, Yee GC, et al., eds. *Pharmacotherapy: A Pathophysiologic Approach.* 8th ed. New York: McGraw-Hill; 2011.

Wilson W, Taubert KA, Gewitz M, et al. Prevention of infective endocarditis: guidelines from the American Heart Association: a guideline from the American Heart Association Rheumatic Fever, Endocarditis, and Kawasaki Disease, Council on Cardiovascular Disease in the Young, and the Council on Clinical Cardiology, Council on Cardiovascular Surgery and Anesthesia, and the Quality of Care and Outcomes Research Interdisciplinary Working Group. *Circulation.* 2007; 116:1736–1754.

II.6 INTRA-ABDOMINAL INFECTIONS

Intra-Abdominal Infections (IAI)		Comments
Definition	**Intra-abdominal infection:** contained within the peritoneal cavity. **Infections of the biliary tract:** • **Cholangitis:** inflammation of the biliary ductal system. • **Cholecystitis:** inflammation of the gallbladder. **Peritonitis:** inflammation of the peritoneal lining. • *Primary:* aka *SBP* or *spontaneous bacterial peritonitis—* develops in the peritoneal cavity without bacterial source within the abdomen. • *Secondary:* fecal contamination within the abdomen caused perforation, postoperative peritonitis, or trauma. • *Tertiary or persistent:* infection that persists or recurs at least 48 hours after initial peritonitis treatment; associated with a higher mortality and morbidity. **Abscesses:** collections of necrotic tissue, bacteria, and white blood cells (WBCs) that form over a period of days to years.	**Primary Peritonitis** • Common in cirrhotic patients; commonly referred to as spontaneous bacterial peritonitis (SBP) • Ascitic fluid positive for leukocytes >300/mm³ and bacteria **Secondary Peritonitis** • Many reasons with appendicitis being most common
	Primary peritonitis: typically caused by a single organism (*E. coli, H. pneumoniae,* Klebsiella, Pseudomonas, anaerobes, and *S. pneumoniae*) **Secondary IAI:** considered polymicrobial; typically enteric gram-negative bacilli and anaerobes	
Common Offending Pathogens	**Gram +:** • *Enterococcus* spp. • *Streptococcus* spp. • *Staphylococcus* spp.	• *S. aureus* most often seen in patients undergoing peritoneal dialysis
	Gram −: • *Enterobacter* spp. • *Escherichia coli* • *Klebsiella pneumoniae* • Proteus	• *E. coli* is most common organism seen in cirrhotic patients with primary peritonitis
	Anaerobes: • *Bacteroides* spp. • *Clostridium* spp. (not *C. difficile*)	• *B. fragilis* is most common anaerobe identified • More common in secondary or tertiary peritonitis

Intra-Abdominal Infections (IAI)			Comments
Common Offending Pathogens	**Fungi:** *Candida* spp.		• If *Candida albicans* **is cultured:** fluconazole is first-line therapy • **For fluconazole-resistant *Candida* spp.:** therapy with an echinocandin (caspofungin, micafungin, anidulafungin) is appropriate • **For critically ill patients:** initial therapy with an echinocandin is recommended
Empiric Treatment of Choice	**Recommended Therapy for Community-Acquired IAIs**		• Early surgical intervention, source control, and adequate drainage is essential for clinical improvement ↑Resistance rates to cefoxitin, especially anaerobes (*B. fragilis*); review site-specific antibiogram
	Type of therapy	**Agent(s) recommended for mild-to-moderate infections**	**Agent(s) recommended for high-severity infections**	
	Single agent			
	Cephalosporin	Cefoxitin 2 g IV Q6h		
	β-lactam/ β-lactamase inhibitor combinations		Piperacillin/tazobactam 4.5 g IV Q6h	
	Carbapenems	Ertapenem 1 g IV Q24h	• Imipenem/ cilastatin 500 mg IV Q6h • Meropenem 1 g IV Q8h • Doripenem 500 mg IV Q8h	
	Glycylcycline	Tigecycline 100 mg IV × 1, then 50 mg IV Q12h		Although FDA-approved, tigecycline not usually first line

Intra-Abdominal Infections (IAI)				Comments
Empiric Treatment of Choice	Type of therapy	Agent(s) recommended for mild-to-moderate infections	Agent(s) recommended for high-severity infections	• Ampicillin-sulbactam not recommended because of high resistance rates to *E. coli*
	Combination regimen			• Cefotetan and clindamycin not recommended because of high resistance rates to *B. fragilis*
	Cephalosporin based	• Cefazolin 2 g IV Q8h plus metronidazole 500 mg IV Q8h • Ceftriaxone 2 g IV Q24h plus metronidazole 500 mg IV Q8h • Cefotaxime 2 g IV Q8h plus metronidazole 500 mg IV Q8h • Cefuroxime 1.5 g IV Q8h plus metronidazole 500 mg IV Q8h	• Ceftazidime 2 g IV Q8h plus metronidazole 500 mg IV Q8h • Cefepime 2 g IV Q8h plus metronidazole 500 mg IV Q8h	• Empiric coverage of Enterococcus and Candida not necessary in community-acquired IAI • **For high-severity, healthcare-acquired infections:** addition of an agent active against gram-positive bacteria such as vancomycin is recommended

	Fluoroquinolone based	• Moxifloxacin 400 mg Q day	• Ciprofloxacin 400 mg IV Q12h plus metronidazole 500 mg IV Q8h
			• Levofloxacin 750 mg IV Q24h plus metronidazole 500 mg IV Q8h
				• **Appendicitis**
				  ○ Antimicrobial therapy should begin prior to the appendectomy
				  ○ Second-generation cephalosporins (cefoxitin)

	Monobactam based		Aztreonam 2 g IV Q8h plus metronidazole 500 mg IV Q8h	

Intra-Abdominal Infections (IAI)			Comments
Empiric Treatment of Choice	**Recommended Therapy for Healthcare IAIs**		○ **Seriously ill:** carbapenem or β-lactam/ β-lactamase inhibitor ○ Post-operative antimicrobial therapy NOT required if appendix was normal or inflamed at time of operation
	Single agent		
	β-lactam/ β-lactamase inhibitor	Piperacillin/tazobactam 4.5 g IV Q6h	
	Carbapenems	• Doripenem 500 mg IV Q8h • Imipenem/cilastatin 500 mg IV Q6h • Meropenem 1 g IV Q8h	
	Combination regimen		
	Cephalosporin based	• Ceftazidime 2 g IV Q8h plus metronidazole 500 mg IV Q8h • Cefepime 2 g IV Q8h plus metronidazole 500 mg IV Q8h	
	Fluoroquinolone based	Ciprofloxacin 400 mg IV Q12h plus metronidazole 500 mg IV Q8h	
	Monobactam based	Aztreonam 2 g IV Q8h plus metronidazole 500 mg IV Q8h	
	Empiric Antifungal Therapy Options: • Anidulafungin 200 mg IV loading dose, then 100 mg IV daily • Caspofungin 70 mg IV loading dose, then 50 mg IV daily • Fluconazole 800 mg × 1, then 400 mg IV Q24h • Micafungin 100 mg IV daily		
Alternative Empiric Treatment Options	For patients with a true type I hypersensitivity reaction to β-lactams: consider aztreonam		
Duration of Therapy	4 to 7 days (may need longer duration of therapy if difficult to achieve source control)		Source control is the key to successful resolution of IAIs. With adequate source control, shorter duration of therapy is recommended (4 days)

REFERENCES

Sawyer RG, Clavidge JA, Nathens AB, et al. Trial of short-course antimicrobial therapy for intra-abdominal infection. *NEJM*. 2015;372:1966–2005.

Solomkin JS, Mazuski JE, Bradley JS, et al. Diagnosis and management of complicated intra-abdominal infection in adults and children: guidelines by the Surgical Infection Society and the Infectious Diseases Society of America. *Clin Infect Dis*. 2010;50:133–164.

II.7   NEUTROPENIC FEVER

Neutropenic Fever		Comments
Definition	• **Fever:** single oral temperature of ≥38.8°C (101°F) or a sustained temperature of ≥38.0°C (100.4°F) over a 1-hour period • **Neutropenia:** ANC <500 cells/mm³ or an ANC that is expected to decrease to <500 cells/mm³ during the next 48 hours • **Profound neutropenia:** ANC <100 cells/mm³ • **High risk:** anticipated prolonged (>7 days duration) and profound neutropenia (ANC <100 cells/mm³) following cytotoxic chemotherapy and/or significant medical comorbid conditions [hypotension, pneumonia, underlying chronic lung disease, new-onset abdominal pain, intravascular catheter infection, oral or gastrointestinal mucositis, neurologic changes, or hepatic (LFTs >5X normal) or renal insufficiency (estimated CrCl <30 mL/min)] • **Low-risk:** anticipated brief (≤7 days duration) neutropenic periods or no or few co-morbidities • **The Multinational Association for Supportive Care in Cancer Risk-Index Score (MASCC):**	Many patients have no identifiable site of infection and no positive cultures. High-risk patients should be admitted to the hospital for empiric antimicrobial therapy (MASCC score <21). Low-risk patients are candidates for oral and/or outpatient empiric antimicrobial therapy (MASCC score ≥21).

Characteristics	Score
Burden of febrile neutropenia with no or mild symptoms[a]	5
No hypotension (systolic blood pressure >90 mmHg)	5
No chronic obstructive pulmonary disease[b]	4
Solid tumor or hematologic malignancy with no previous fungal infection[c]	4
No dehydration requiring parenteral fluids	3
Burden of febrile neutropenia with moderate symptoms	3
Outpatient status	3
Age <60 years	2

Maximum value of the score is 26.

[a] Burden of febrile neutropenia refers to the general clinical status of the patient as influenced by the febrile neutropenic episode. Should be evaluated on the following scale: no or mild symptoms (score of 5); moderate symptoms (score of 3); and severe symptoms or moribund (score of 0).

[b] Chronic obstructive pulmonary disease means active chronic bronchitis, emphysema, decrease in forced expiratory volumes, need for oxygen therapy and/or steroids and/or bronchodilators requiring treatment at the presentation of the febrile neutropenic episode.

[c] Previous fungal infection means demonstrated fungal infection or empirically treated suspected fungal infection.

	Neutropenic Fever	Comments
Common Offending Pathogens	**Gram +:** Coagulase-negative staphylococci *Enterococcus* spp. (including VRE) *Staphylococcus aureus* (including MRSA) *Streptococcus pneumoniae* *Streptococcus pyogenes* Viridans group streptococci	Coagulase-negative staphylococci is the most common cause of bacteremia in neutropenic patients. Careful assessment if only 1 out of ≥2 blood cultures as it may still be contaminant.
	Gram −: *Acinetobacter* spp. *Citrobacter* spp. *Enterobacter* spp. *Escherichia coli* *Klebsiella* spp. *Pseudomonas aeruginosa* *Stenotrophomonas maltophilia*	May be extended-spectrum β-lactamase (ESBL) producing or carbapenemase-resistant *Enterobacteriaceae* (CRE), specifically *Klebsiella pneumoniae* carbapenemase (KPC)
	Yeast: *Candida* spp.	Colonize mucosal surfaces
	Mold: *Aspergillus*	May cause infection in the sinuses and/or lungs; typically after ≥2 weeks of neutropenia
Empiric Treatment of Choice	<u>**High Risk:**</u> **Antipseudomonal β-lactam monotherapy** (e.g., cefepime, ceftazidime, piperacillin/tazobactam, carbapenems)	Other antimicrobials (e.g., aminoglycosides, fluoroquinolones, and/or vancomycin) may be added to the initial regimen for management of complications (e.g., hypotension and pneumonia) or if antimicrobial resistance is suspected/proven

Neutropenic Fever		Comments
Empiric Treatment of Choice	<u>For:</u> **ESBL:** Consider early use of a carbapenem **KPCs/CREs:** Consider early use of colistin or tigecycline (avoid if bloodstream infections) **MRSA:** Consider early addition of vancomycin, linezolid, daptomycin, or ceftaroline **VRE:** Consider early addition of linezolid or daptomycin	Vancomycin (or other gram + agents) is not recommended as part of the initial antimicrobial regimen. Consider for specific clinical indications (suspected catheter-related infections, skin and soft tissue infections, pneumonia, hemodynamic instability, or positive blood culture with gram + organisms) Empiric antifungal therapy should be considered in patients who have persistent neutropenic fever despite 4–7 days of empiric antimicrobial therapy; avoid fluconazole in patients who received fluconazole prophylaxis Antimicrobial changes or additions to the initial empiric regimen should be based on clinical, radiographic, or microbiological evidence of infection and not on the persistence of fever alone in a patient whose condition is otherwise stable

Neutropenic Fever		Comments
Empiric Treatment of Choice	<u>Low Risk:</u> Ciprofloxacin plus amoxicillin/clavulanate (also levofloxacin or ciprofloxacin as monotherapy or ciprofloxacin plus clindamycin)	Low-risk patients should receive initial oral or IV therapy in a clinic or hospital setting and may be transitioned to outpatient oral or IV therapy if specific criteria are met
		Patient should be able to tolerate and absorb oral antimicrobials
		Patients who are receiving fluoroquinolone prophylaxis should not receive oral empiric fluoroquinolone therapy
		Patients should be admitted for persistent fever or signs and symptoms of worsening infection
Alternative Empiric Treatment Options	For patients with a true type I hypersensitivity reaction to β-lactams, consider cefepime or carbapenem or aztreonam for gram-negative coverage (including *Pseudomonas*) plus vancomycin or ciprofloxacin plus clindamycin	
Duration of Therapy	In patients with clinically or microbiologically documented infections, duration of antimicrobial therapy depends on the particular organism and site; appropriate antimicrobials should continue for at least the duration of neutropenia (until ANC >500 cells/mm^3) or longer if clinically necessary. In patients with unexplained fever, the initial regimen should be continued until there are clear signs of marrow recovery (increasing ANC >500 cells/mm^3). Alternatively, if an appropriate treatment course has been completed and all signs and symptoms of a documented infection have resolved, patients who remain neutropenic may resume oral fluoroquinolone prophylaxis until marrow recovery.	

REFERENCE

Freifeld AG, Bow EJ, Sepkowitz KA, et al. Clinical practice guideline for the use of antimicrobial agents in neutropenic patients with cancer: 2010 update by the Infectious Diseases Society of America. *Clin Infect Dis.* 2011;52:e56–e93.

❖ ❖ ❖

II.8   OTITIS MEDIA

	Otitis Media	Comments
Definition	**Otitis Media (OM):** inflammation of the middle ear. Usually follows a viral upper respiratory infection that causes eustachian tube dysfunction and mucosal swelling in the middle ear **Symptoms include:** • Fever • Ear pain • Tugging on the ear • Irritability • Difficulty sleeping • Gray, bulging limited or nonmotile tympanic membrane (TM) • Air-fluid level behind the TM • Discharge from the ear • Children may also experience rhinorrhea, nasal congestion, or cough in the days preceding OM symptoms **Complications of OM are infrequent but include:** mastoiditis, bacteremia, meningitis, hearing loss that may lead to speech and language developmental delays	Children are more susceptible than adults because the anatomy of their eustachian tube is shorter and more horizontal, which then facilitates bacterial entry into the middle ear **Risk factors for the development of OM include:** • Daycare setting • Lack of breastfeeding • Pacifier use • Early age of first diagnosis • Nasopharyngeal colonization • Siblings in the home • Lower socioeconomic status • Male gender • Allergy • Exposure to cigarette smoke urban population immunodeficiency
Deciding to Treat	• Up to 80% of OM cases resolve spontaneously without intervention • If observation off antimicrobials is selected, close follow-up is recommended	

Age	Confirmed Diagnosis	Uncertain Diagnosis
6 months	Antimicrobials recommended	Antimicrobials recommended
6 months to 2 years	Antimicrobials recommended	Severe illness:[†] antimicrobials recommended Non-severe illness:[§] Observation off antimicrobials

Key: *Less frequently encountered pathogens; † severe illness: moderate-to-severe ear pain or fever ≥102.6° F; §non-severe illness: mild ear pain and fever <102.6° F

Otitis Media			Comments
Deciding to Treat	**Age**	**Confirmed Diagnosis**	**Uncertain Diagnosis**
	≥2 years	Severe illness: antimicrobials recommended[†] Non-severe illness: Observation off antimicrobials[§]	Observation
Common Offending Pathogens	Viruses (~45%) *Streptococcus pneumoniae* (20–35%) *Haemophilus influenzae* *Moraxella catarrhalis* *Staphylococcus aureus** *Streptococcus pyogenes** Gram-negative bacilli (such as *Pseudomonas aeruginosa*)*		
Empiric Treatment *Pediatric doses listed	**First Line:** • Amoxicillin (80–90 mg/kg/day divided Q12h)		**Treatment Failure** • Amoxicillin-clavulanate (90 mg/kg/day PO Q12h) • Ceftriaxone (50 mg/kg/day IM or IV for 3 days)
	If severe symptoms (severe ear pain and fever ≥102.6° F) • Amoxicillin-clavulanate (80–90 mg/kg/day divided Q12h)		**Treatment Failure** • Clindamycin (30–40 mg/kg/day divided Q8h)
	Mild β-lactam allergy • Cefdinir (14 mg/kg/day or divided Q12h) • Cefuroxime (30 mg/kg/day divided Q12h) • Cefpodoxime (10 mg/kg/day) • Cefprozil (30 mg/kg/day divided Q12h)		**Mild allergy:** erythematous, non-pruritic, rash
	Severe β-lactam allergy • Azithromycin (10 mg/kg/day 1, then 5 mg/kg/day days 2–5) • Clarithromycin (15 mg/kg/day divided Q12h)		**Severe allergy:** anaphylaxis, angioedema, urticaria
Supportive Therapy	• Acetaminophen or ibuprofen for pain and fever • Tympanostomy tubes for prevention may be considered in the following: ○ >3 OM episodes in 6 months or ○ ≥4 OM episodes in a year		
Duration of Therapy	Patients <5 years old and children with severe disease = 10 days Patients ≥6 years with mild-to-moderate OM = 5–7 days		

REFERENCE

American Academy of Pediatrics Subcommittee on Management of Acute Otits Media: Diagnosis and management of acute otitis media. *Pediatrics.* 2004;113:1451–1465.

II.9 PHARYNGITIS

	Pharyngitis	Comments
Definition	**Pharyngitis:** Infection of the oropharynx or nasopharynx **Symptoms include:** • Sore throat with rapid, sudden onset • Pain on swallowing • Fever • Redness and swelling of the tonsils and pharynx • Enlarged, tender lymph nodes • Red swollen uvula • Petechiae on the soft palate • Scarlatiniform rash **Children may also experience:** • Headache • Nausea • Vomiting • Abdominal pain	Seasonal outbreaks common especially in winter and early spring If Group A *Streptococcus* (GAS) patients are left untreated, they can be contagious for up to a week after the acute illness; antimicrobials reduce the infectious period to 24 hours GAS rarely causes pharyngitis in children <3 years of age **Complications:** • Acute glomerulonephritis • Acute rheumatic fever • Cervical lymphadenitis mastoiditis • Necrotizing fasciitis • Otitis media • Peritonsillar abscess • Reactive arthritis • Retropharyngeal abscess • Sinusitis **Risk factors:** • Children ages 5–15 years old • Parents of school-age children • Those who work with children
Common Offending Pathogens	Viruses *Streptococcus pyogenes* (GAS) **Other less likely organisms:*** *Streptococcus* spp. *Arcanobacterium haemolyticum* *Corynebacterium diphtheriae* *Neisseria gonorrhea* *Mycoplasma pneumoniae* Anaerobes *Fusobacterium necrophorum* *Do not require antimicrobial therapy	"Strep throat" is difficult to differentiate from viral pharyngitis. Due to this diagnostic challenge, swabbing the throat and testing for GAS pharyngitis using rapid antigen detection and/or culture should be performed. If the rapid antigen testing is negative in children and adolescents, results should be confirmed with a throat culture; however, if a positive rapid antigen test is positive, there is no need to confirm with culture. A common misperception is that the "rapid strep test" tests for *S. pneumoniae*; however, it actually tests for GAS.
Treatment for GAS	**Children:** • Penicillin VK (50 mg/kg/day PO divided Q8h) • Amoxicillin (50 mg/kg/day PO divided Q8h) • Penicillin benzathine (<27 kg 0.6 million units IM; ≥27 kg 1.2 million units IM)	**β-Lactam Allergy** Children: • Cephalexin (20 mg/kg/dose PO Q12h) • Cefadroxil (30 mg/kg PO daily) • Clindamycin (7 mg/kg/dose PO Q8h) • Azithromycin (12 mg/kg PO daily) • Clarithromycin (7.5 mg/kg/dose PO Q12h)

Pharyngitis		Comments
Treatment for GAS	**Adults:** • Penicillin VK (250 mg PO Q6h or 500 mg PO Q12h) • Amoxicillin (500 mg PO Q8h) • Penicillin benzathine (1.2 million units IM)	<u>Adults:</u> • Cephalexin (500 mg PO Q12h) • Cefadroxil (1,000 mg PO daily) • Clindamycin (300 mg PO Q8h) • Azithromycin (500 mg × 1 dose then 250 mg daily × 5 days) • Clarithromycin (250–500 mg PO Q12h)
Supportive Therapy	Acetaminophen (APAP) or ibuprofen may be used to relieve pain (however, APAP preferred due to the risk for necrotizing fasciitis and toxic shock syndrome) Rest, fluids, lozenges, and saltwater gargles may be encouraged	
Duration of Therapy	10 days	

REFERENCE

Shulman ST, Bisno AL, Clegg HW, et al. Clinical practice guidelines for the diagnosis and management of group A streptococcal pharyngitis: 2012 update by the Infectious Diseases Society of America. *Clin Infect Dis.* 2012;55:1279–1282.

II.10 PNEUMONIA

II.10.1 COMMUNITY-ACQUIRED PNEUMONIA IN ADULTS

Community-Acquired Pneumonia (CAP)		Comments
Definitions	**Community-Acquired Pneumonia (CAP):** Pneumonia that occurs in patients presenting from a community setting without any healthcare-associated risk factors.	CAP affects patients of all ages and may occur at any time of the year. Clinical manifestations tend to be more severe in the very young, the elderly, and patients who are immunocompromised.
Common Offending Pathogens	**Gram +:** *Streptococcus pneumoniae* *Staphylococcus aureus*	*Streptococcus pneumoniae* is the most common pathogen *Staphylococcus aureus* is uncommon; usually results in severe pneumonia
	Gram −: *Haemophilus influenzae* *Moraxella catarrhalis* *Klebsiella pneumoniae* (alcoholism) *Pseudomonas aeruginosa* Other gram-negative bacilli	Pseudomonas risk factors below.

Community-Acquired Pneumonia (CAP)		Comments
Common Offending Pathogens	**Anaerobes:** Uncommon	Usually only seen with aspiration
	Atypicals: *Chlamydophila pneumoniae* *Legionella* spp. *Mycoplasma pneumoniae*	*Mycoplasma pneumoniae* and *Chlamydophila pneumoniae* typically cause less severe pneumonia Patients with *Legionella* typically require ICU admission
	Respiratory viruses: Influenza A and B, parainfluenza, adenovirus, and respiratory syncytial virus	No antiviral treatment except for influenza: • Oseltamivir (adults 75 mg PO Q12h × 5 days; children ≤15 kg 30 mg Q12h, 16–23 kg 45 mg Q12h, 24–40 kg 60 mg Q12h, ≥41 kg 75 mg Q12h × 5 days) • Zanamivir (adults and children ≥7 years old 2 puffs [5 mg/puff] Q12h)
Empiric Treatment	**Outpatient:** For previously healthy patients with no risk factors for drug-resistant *Streptococcus pneumoniae:* • Macrolide • Doxycycline	**Macrolides:** • Azithromycin 500 mg PO × 1 then 250 mg daily × 4 days or 500 mg daily × 3 days **Other:** • Doxycycline 100 mg PO Q12h
	For patients with any of the following comorbidities: Chronic renal, hepatic, heart, or lung disease, diabetes mellitus, alcoholism, malignancies, asplenia, immunosuppressing conditions or current use of immunosuppressing medications: or Use of antimicrobials within previous 90 days, or other risk factors for drug-resistant *Streptococcus pneumoniae*, or in areas with >25% of infections with high level macrolide-resistant *S. pneumoniae:* • Respiratory fluoroquinolone • β-lactam plus macrolide (or doxycycline for patients with macrolide allergy/intolerance, or concern for drug interactions or adverse effects such as QT prolongation)	**Respiratory fluoroquinolones:*** • Moxifloxacin 400 mg daily • Levofloxacin 750 mg daily *Ciprofloxacin is not considered a respiratory fluoroquinolone due to the lack of *S. pneumoniae* coverage; has excellent lung penetration **β-lactams (preferred):** • Amoxicillin 1 g Q8h • Amoxicillin/clavulanate 875 mg Q12h or ER tab 2 g Q12h • Ceftriaxone 1 g Q24h (2 g if patient ≥100 kg) • Cefpodoxime 200 mg Q12h • Cefuroxime 500 mg Q12h The combination of β-lactam and macrolide is used due to ↑ resistance with *S. pneumoniae* and macrolides. Therefore, β-lactams are used for their *S. pneumoniae* coverage whereas the macrolides provide atypical coverage

Community-Acquired Pneumonia (CAP)		Comments
Empiric Treatment	**Inpatient, Non-ICU:** • Respiratory fluoroquinolone • β-lactam plus macrolide For multiple documented concomitant severe penicillin and cephalosporin allergies and fluoroquinolone allergy or potential fluoroquinolone drug interaction or adverse effect concern may consider: • Tigecycline 100 mg × 1 then 50 mg Q12h	Consider previous antimicrobial therapy when selecting empiric antimicrobials (i.e., if a patient was receiving a β-lactam or a macrolide prior to admission, consider a respiratory fluoroquinolone or if a patient was receiving a fluoroquinolone prior to admission, consider a β-lactam plus macrolide, etc.) **β-lactams (preferred):** • Ceftriaxone 1 g IV Q24h (2 g if patient ≥100 kg) • Cefotaxime 1 g IV Q8h (2 g if patient >80 kg) • Ampicillin/sulbactam 1.5 g IV Q6h (3 g if patient >80 kg) • Ertapenem 1 g IV Q24h
	Inpatient, ICU: • β-lactam plus macrolide (intravenous formulation) • β-lactam plus respiratory fluoroquinolone (intravenous formulation) For multiple documented concomitant severe penicillin and cephalosporin allergies: • Respiratory fluoroquinolone	**β-lactams (preferred):** • Ceftriaxone 1 g Q24h (2 g if patient ≥100 kg) • Cefotaxime 1 g Q8h (2 g if patient >80 kg) • Ampicillin-sulbactam 1.5 g Q6h (3 g if patient >80 kg) The IV formulation of the selected macrolide or respiratory fluoroquinolone is utilized in initial therapy due to possible reduced GI absorption of oral medications in hypotensive patients
	Pseudomonas risk: • Antipseudomonal β-lactam plus fluoroquinolone or macrolide For multiple documented concomitant severe penicillin and cephalosporin allergies: • Aztreonam plus antipneumococcal fluoroquinolone plus consider the addition of 24–48 hours of aminoglycosides depending on severity of illness, history of MDRO, and local antibiogram	Pseudomonas risk includes patients with **either:** • Bronchiectasis or • Structural lung disease (chronic bronchitis, COPD, emphysema, interstitial lung disease, pulmonary fibrosis) plus either chronic systemic steroids or a history of repeated (multiple courses) antimicrobial use. • Chronic steroid or repeated antimicrobial use can be for any reason; it does not have to be linked to the structural lung disease.

Community-Acquired Pneumonia (CAP)		Comments
Duration of Therapy	5–7 days	Patients should be afebrile for 48–72 hours and should show signs of clinical improvement before discontinuation of antimicrobials
		Longer duration may be needed if initial therapy was not active against identified pathogen
Other Comments	Influenza vaccine, pneumococcal vaccine, and smoking cessation counseling should be offered to patients.	

REFERENCE

Mandell LA, Wunderink RG, Anzueto A, et al. Infectious Diseases Society of America/American Thoracic Society consensus guidelines on the management of community-acquired pneumonia in adults. *Clin Infect Dis.* 2007;44:S27–72.

II.10.2 COMMUNITY-ACQUIRED PNEUMONIA IN CHILDREN

Patient Location/Age	Common Pathogens	Treatment Recommendations for Presumed Bacterial CAP	Treatment Recommendations for Presumed Atypical CAP	Treatment for Presumed Viral CAP
Outpatient				
<5 years (preschool)	• Viruses: ○ RSV ○ Parainfluenza virus ○ Influenza ○ Adenovirus ○ Metapneumovirus • *Streptococcus pneumoniae* • *Haemophilus pneumoniae*	Amoxicillin (90 mg/kg/day PO divided Q12h) **Alternative:** Amoxicillin-clavulanate (amoxicillin component 90 mg/kg/day PO divided Q12h)	Azithromycin (10 mg/kg PO on day 1, then 5 mg/kg/day days 2–5) **Alternatives:** Clarithromycin (15 mg/kg/day PO divided Q12h) or Erythromycin (40 mg/kg/day PO divided Q6h)	No antimicrobials recommended for viruses; supportive care only **If influenza:** Oseltamivir (children ≤15 kg 30 mg Q12h, 16–23 kg 45 mg Q12h, 24–40 kg 60 mg Q12h, ≥41 kg 75 mg Q12h × 5 days)

Patient Location/Age	Common Pathogens	Treatment Recommendations for Presumed Bacterial CAP	Treatment Recommendations for Presumed Atypical CAP	Treatment for Presumed Viral CAP
Outpatient				
≥5 years	Consider atypical organisms: • *Chlamydophila pneumoniae* • *Mycoplasma pneumoniae*	Amoxicillin (90 mg/kg/day PO divided Q12h; maximum of 4 g/day) **If atypical infection cannot be ruled out: ADD** azithromycin (10 mg/kg PO on day 1, then 5 mg/kg/day days 2–5) **Alternative:** Amoxicillin-clavulanate (amoxicillin component 90 mg/kg/day PO divided Q12h; maximum of 4 g/day)	Azithromycin (10 mg/kg PO on day 1, then 5 mg/kg/day days 2–5; maximum of 500 mg on day 1 and 250 mg on days 2–5) **Alternatives:** Clarithromycin (15 mg/kg/day PO divided Q12h; maximum of 1 g/day) or Erythromycin (40 mg/kg/day PO divided Q6h) or Doxycycline for children >7 years old	**If influenza:** Oseltamivir (dosing as above) or Zanamivir (children ≥7 years old, 2 puffs [5 mg/puff] Q12h)
Inpatient (all ages) <18 years				
Fully immunized with conjugate vaccines for *Haemophilus pneumoniae* type b and ***Streptococcus pneumoniae*; local penicillin resistance in pneumococcus minimal**	• *Chlamydophila pneumoniae* • *Haemophilus pneumoniae* • *Mycoplasma pneumoniae* • *Streptococcus pneumoniae*	Ampicillin or penicillin G **Alternatives:** Ceftriaxone or cefotaxime Addition of vancomycin or clindamycin for suspected community-acquired MRSA	Azithromycin in addition to ceftriaxone or cefotaxime (if atypical not confirmed) **Alternatives:** Clarithromycin (15 mg/kg/day PO divided Q12h; maximum of 1 g/day) or Erythromycin (40 mg/kg/day PO divided Q6h) or	**If influenza:** Oseltamivir or Zanamivir (children >7 years old)

Patient Location/Age	Common Pathogens	Treatment Recommendations for Presumed Bacterial CAP	Treatment Recommendations for Presumed Atypical CAP	Treatment for Presumed Viral CAP
Inpatient (all ages) <18 years				
Not fully immunized with conjugate vaccines for *Haemophilus pneumoniae* type b and *Streptococcus pneumoniae*; local penicillin resistance in pneumococcus significant		Ceftriaxone or cefotaxime Addition of vancomycin or clindamycin for suspected community-acquired MRSA **Alternatives:** Levofloxacin Addition of vancomycin or clindamycin for suspected community-acquired MRSA	doxycycline for children >7 years old Levofloxacin for children who have reached growth maturity who cannot tolerate macrolides Azithromycin in addition to ceftriaxone or cefotaxime (if atypical not confirmed)	

REFERENCE

Bradley JS, Byington CL, Shah SS, et al. The management of community-acquired pneumonia in infants and children older than 3 months of age: clinical practice guidelines by the Pediatric Infectious Diseases Society and the Infectious Diseases Society of America. *Clin Infect Dis.* 2011;53:e25–e76.

II.10.3   HEALTHCARE-ASSOCIATED PNEUMONIA

Healthcare-Associated Pneumonia (Includes Healthcare-Associated Pneumonia [HCAP], Hospital-Acquired Pneumonia [HAP], and Ventilator-Associated Pneumonia [VAP])		Comments
Definitions	Healthcare-Associated Pneumonia (HCAP): Pneumonia that occurs in a patient who has any of the following risk factors: • Hospitalization for ≥48 hours within 90 days • Residence in a nursing home or extended care facility • Antimicrobial use within 30 days • Home infusion therapy (e.g., antimicrobials, chemotherapy, etc.) or home wound care	**Low risk for multidrug-resistant organisms (MDROs):** • **Early onset**—occurs within the first 4 days of hospitalization **High risk for MDROs:** • **Late onset**—occurs after ≥5 days of hospitalization

Healthcare-Associated Pneumonia (Includes Healthcare-Associated Pneumonia [HCAP], Hospital-Acquired Pneumonia [HAP], and Ventilator-Associated Pneumonia [VAP])		Comments
Definitions	• Chronic dialysis within 30 days • Family member with multidrug-resistant pathogens **Hospital-Acquired Pneumonia (HAP):** Pneumonia that occurs ≥48 hours after hospital admission and not incubating at time of admission. **Ventilator-Associated Pneumonia (VAP):** Pneumonia that occurs >48–72 hours after endotracheal intubation.	• Antimicrobial therapy within the last 90 days (consider broad spectrum, multiple courses, etc.) • High frequency of antimicrobial resistance in the community or hospital unit • Immunosuppressive disease and/or therapy • History of infection or colonization with a multidrug-resistant organism • Any of the HCAP risk factors listed on the previous page
Common Offending Pathogens	**Gram +:** Methicillin-resistant *Staphylococcus aureus* (MRSA) *Streptococcus pneumoniae* (early-onset only)	MRSA more common in patients with diabetes mellitus, head trauma, ICU admission, and ventilated patients For MRSA, consider local prevalence
	Gram −: *Acinetobacter* spp. *Citrobacter* spp. *Enterobacter* spp. *Escherichia coli* *Haemophilus influenzae* (early onset only) *Klebsiella pneumoniae* *Pseudomonas aeruginosa* *Serratia* spp. *Stenotrophomonas maltophilia*	*Enterobacter, Citrobacter,* and *Serratia* have an inducible chromosomal AmpC β-lactamase; if isolated, consider cefepime or carbapenem use *Pseudomonas, Acinetobacter,* and *Stenotrophomonas* are common colonizers of respiratory tract in ventilated patients
	Anaerobes: Uncommon cause of VAP	May be associated with aspiration in nonventilated patients
	Atypicals: *Legionella pneumophila*	Incidence is variable, increased incidence in immunocompromised patients (e.g., organ transplant, HIV, diabetes mellitus, underlying lung disease, or end-stage renal disease, etc.) More common when present in hospital water supply or during construction; consider local prevalence

Healthcare-Associated Pneumonia (Includes Healthcare-Associated Pneumonia [HCAP], Hospital-Acquired Pneumonia [HAP], and Ventilator-Associated Pneumonia [VAP])	Comments
Empiric Treatment of Choice	**Antipseudomonal β-lactam** (e.g., cefepime, ceftazidime, piperacillin/tazobactam, imipenem, meropenem, or doripenem) +/− **Antipseudomonal fluoroquinolone** (e.g., ciprofloxacin, levofloxacin) or **Aminoglycoside** (e.g., amikacin, gentamicin, tobramycin) +/− **Glycopeptide** or **oxazolidinone** (e.g., vancomycin or linezolid)	Not all patients require MRSA coverage. Consider in patients with a history of MRSA infections, MRSA colonization (nasal/throat) status, and critically ill with sepsis or ICU admission. Also consider hospital incidence of MRSA. If empiric double gram negative coverage, consider deescalation once patient stabilizes and/or culture data are available
Alternative Empiric Treatment Options	For patients with a true type I hypersensitivity reaction to β-lactams, may consider aztreonam for gram-negative coverage including *Pseudomonas* although concern for increasing resistance. Careful consideration of allergy history to confirm true allergy. Patients with history of type I hypersensitivity may tolerate some cephalosporins or carbapenems. IgE antibodies to PCN wane over time (i.e., patients with true allergic reaction early in life may be able to tolerate PCN later)—validated in studies with PCN skin testing and through observational studies.	
Duration of Therapy	7 to 8 days 14 days for patients with nonfermenting gram-negative pathogens (e.g., *Pseudomonas, Acinetobacter*, etc.)	

REFERENCE

American Thoracic Society, Infectious Diseases Society of America. Guidelines for the management of adults with hospital-acquired, ventilator-associated, and healthcare-associated pneumonia. *Am J Respir Crit Care Med.* 2005;171:388–416.

II.11   RHINOSINUSITIS

	Rhinosinusitis	Comments
Definitions	**Rhinosinusitis or sinusitis:** an inflammation and/or infection of the lining of the nasal passages and paranasal sinus mucosa. **Symptoms include:** • Ear pressure/pain • Headache • Laryngitis (chronic sinusitis) • Nasal congestion • Nonproductive cough • Rhinorrhea • Tooth, facial, or sinus pain/pressure	Antimicrobial over-prescribing is a major concern in the management of acute sinusitis, largely due to the difficulty in differentiating between bacterial sinusitis and viral sinusitis. This is due to the similar presentation, and it is difficult and/or painful to obtain cultures. Viral infections usually resolve on their own within 7–10 days. If symptoms persist longer than this or worsen, it is likely bacterial and requires antimicrobial therapy. High fevers (≥39°C) or severe pain (≥3–4 days) may be associated with bacterial sinusitis as well. Bacterial sinusitis may persist for 4 weeks and may become chronic (>3 months).
Common Offending Pathogens	Viruses *Haemophilus influenzae* *Moraxella catarrhalis* *Staphylococcus aureus** *Streptococcus pneumoniae* *Streptococcus pyogenes** Anaerobes* Fungi* ──── *Much less frequent pathogens	
Initial Treatment Once Bacterial Source Confirmed	**FIRST-LINE** **Children:** Amoxicillin-clavulanate (45 mg/kg/day PO Q12h)	**SECOND-LINE** **Children:** Amoxicillin-clavulanate (90 mg/kg/day PO Q12h)
	FIRST-LINE **Adults:** Amoxicillin-clavulanate (500/125 mg PO Q8h or 875/125 mg PO Q12h)	**SECOND-LINE** **Adults:** • Amoxicillin-clavulanate ER tabs (2,000/125 mg PO Q12h) • Doxycycline (100 mg PO Q12h or 200 mg PO daily)

	Rhinosinusitis	Comments
β-Lactam Allergy	**Children:** *Mild allergy* Clindamycin (30–40 mg/kg/day PO Q8h) plus cefixime (8 mg/kg/day PO Q12h) or cefpodoxime (10 mg/kg/day PO Q12h) *Severe allergy* Levofloxacin (10–20 mg/kg/day PO Q12–24h)	*Mild allergy:* erythemateous, non-pruritic, rash *Severe allergy:* anaphylaxis, angioedema, urticaria
	Adults: • Doxycycline (100 mg PO Q12h or 200 mg PO daily) • Levofloxacin (500 mg PO daily) • Moxifloxacin (400 mg PO daily)	
Risk for Antimicrobial Resistance or Failed Initial Therapy	**Children:** • Amoxicillin-clavulanate (90 mg/kg/day PO Q12h) • Clindamycin (30–40 mg/kg/day PO Q8h) plus cefixime (8 mg/kg/day PO Q12h) or cefpodoxime (10 mg/kg/day PO Q12h) • Levofloxacin (10–20 mg/kg/day PO Q12–24h)	Factors associated with antimicrobial resistance include: age <2 or >65, daycare, prior antibiotics within the past 3 months or hospitalization in the past 5 days, comorbidities, and immunocompromised state.
	Adults: • Amoxicillin-clavulanate (2,000/125 mg PO Q12h) • Levofloxacin (500 mg PO daily) • Moxifloxacin (400 mg PO daily)	
Severe Infection Requiring Hospitalization	**Children:** • Ampicillin-sulbactam (200–400 mg/kg/day IV Q6h) • Ceftriaxone (50 mg/kg/day IV Q12h) • Cefotaxime (100–200 mg/kg/day IV Q6h) • Levofloxacin (10–20 mg/kg/day PO Q12–24h)	Uncommon for patients to require hospitalization
	Adults: • Ampicillin-sulbactam (1.5–3 g IV Q6h) • Cefotaxime (2 g IV Q4–6h) • Ceftriaxone (1–2 g IV Q24h) • Levofloxacin (500 mg PO or IV daily) • Moxifloxacin (400 mg PO or IV daily)	
Supportive Therapy	• Analgesics for sinus pain, headache, or fever • Avoid antihistamines as they can dry nasal mucosa and disturb the clearance of mucosal secretions • Decongestants may slightly relieve symptoms; however, are associated with risks (e.g., adverse effects, rebound congestion with topical decongestant use >3 days) and should be avoided in children	

	Rhinosinusitis	Comments
Supportive Therapy	• Intranasal corticosteroids may be considered, especially in those with allergic rhinitis as they reduce mucosal swelling and promote drainage • Saline irrigation is also recommended as it has been shown to provide symptomatic relief, is inexpensive, and is safe (may cause nasal burning or irritation)	
Duration of Therapy	5–7 days in adults and 10–14 days in children	

REFERENCE

Chow AW, Benninger MS, Brook I, et al. IDSA Clinical practice guideline for acute bacterial rhinosinusitis in children and adults. *Clin Infect Dis.* 2012;54:e72–e112.

II.12   SEPSIS AND SEPTIC SHOCK IN ADULTS

	Sepsis and Septic Shock	Comments
Definitions	**SIRS**—systemic inflammatory response syndrome (may or may not be due to infection) **Sepsis**—the presence (probable or documented) of infection together with systemic manifestations of infection (≥2 SIRS criteria) **Severe sepsis**—sepsis plus sepsis-induced tissue hypoperfusion or organ dysfunction **Septic shock**—sepsis-induced hypotension persisting despite adequate fluid resuscitation resulting from marked reduction in systemic vascular resistance **Multiple organ dysfunction syndrome (MODS)**—progressive organ dysfunction in an acutely ill patient such that homeostasis cannot be maintained without intervention	**SIRS Criteria** • Temperature >38°C (100.4°F) or <36°C (96.8°F) • Heart rate >90 bpm • Respiratory rate >20 or $PaCO_2$ <32 mmHg • WBC >12,000 cells/mm³, <4,000 cells/mm³, or 10% bands **Organ Dysfunction Criteria** • Urine output < 0.5 mL/kg/hr despite fluids • SCr increases > 0.5 mg/dL • Coagulation abnormalities (INR > 1.5 or aPTT > 60 sec); consider anticoagulation therapy • Ileus (bowel sounds absent) • Thrombocytopenia • Hyperbilirubinemia (>4 mg/dL) • Tissue perfusion • Hyperlactatemia • Decreased capillary refill or mottling

	Sepsis and Septic Shock	Comments
Initial Resuscitation	• Lactate (**baseline and repeated within 6 hours of onset if initial lactate was elevated**) • Obtain blood cultures prior to antimicrobial therapy • Other pertinent cultures (urine, sputum, etc.) and imaging to confirm infection	**Goals:** CVP 8–12 mmHg; MAP ≥65 mmHg Urine output ≥0.5 mL/kg/hr Central venous (superior vena cava) or mixed oxygen saturation 70% or 65%, respectively Normalize lactate **Blood cultures:** at least **2 sets** of blood cultures from **two different sites** (administration of antimicrobials should **NOT** be delayed if blood cultures cannot be obtained)
IV Fluids	• Fluid resuscitation (30 mL/kg) crystalloid for hypotension or lactate ≥4 mmol/L • Start maintenance fluids • Assess fluid responsiveness (see comments)	Methods to assess fluid responsiveness include all five of the following: vital signs, cadiopulmonary exam, capillary refill evaluation, peripheral pulse evaluation, and skin examination or CVP monitoring, SvO_2 measurement, bedside cardiovascular ultrasound, passive leg raise, or fluid challenge Usually a one-time bolus in a fluid-restricted patient with sepsis is OK; adjust maintenance in these patients **Goals:** CVP 8–12 mmHg or 12–15 mmHg for mechanically ventilated patients
Empiric Antimicrobial Therapy	Initiate appropriate empiric broad spectrum therapy based on the suspected site of infection **within 1 hour** of sepsis recognition or suspicion. As per CMS recommendations, patients should receive monotherapy with any of the agents listed on next page on the left or combination therapy with two agents on the right for the management of sepsis within 3 hours of symptom onset.	Every hour delay of antimicrobials results in 7.6% increase in mortality. Choosing incorrect initial antimicrobial increases mortality by 50%.

Sepsis and Septic Shock			Comments
Empiric Antimicrobial Therapy	**CMS Acceptable Antimicrobials for Sepsis**		Antimicrobial selection should be based on suspected site and severity of infection, hospital empiric use guidelines, local susceptibility patterns, and some patient-specific factors such as allergies, healthcare-associated risk factors, comorbidities, organ dysfunction, immune status, weight, etc.
	Monotherapy	**Combination Therapy**	
	Carbapenems • Meropenem • Imipenem/ Cilastatin • Doripenem • Ertapenem **Cephalosporins** • Cefotaxime • Ceftriaxone • Ceftazidime • Cefepime • Ceftaroline **Fluoroquinolones** • Moxifloxacin • Levofloxacin **Penicillins** • Piperacillin/ Tazobactam • Ampicillin/ Sulbactam	Aminoglycosides or Aztreonam or Ciprofloxacin plus Cephalosporins (first-and second-generation) or Clindamycin (IV) or Daptomycin or Vancomycin or Linezolid or Macrolides or Penicillins	Antimicrobial therapy should be assessed daily for de-escalation opportunities Combination therapy increases the likelihood that at least one drug is effective and is associated with superior outcomes in severely ill, septic patients with a high mortality risk Specific examples of patient populations in whom combination therapy may be most beneficial include (but not limited to): • Neutropenic patients with severe sepsis • Infections caused by multidrug-resistant organisms (MDROs) or empirically for patients at high risk of MDRO • Severe infection associated with respiratory failure and septic shock
	Careful consideration of the site of infection should be determined. If sepsis of unknown etiology, broad spectrum therapy should be administered to cover all potential pathogens. Procalcitonin levels may be beneficial to de-escalate or discontinue therapy.		If combination antimicrobial therapy is initiated, **careful consideration of the sequence of administration should be performed** (e.g., if piperacillin/ tazobactam and vancomycin are initiated, administer piperacillin/tazobactam [broad spectrum] first followed by the vancomycin); **GIVE BROAD SPECTRUM FIRST** • Consider line access, drug compatibilities, and suspected source of infection

	Sepsis and Septic Shock	Comments
Empiric Antimicrobial Therapy		Routine empiric antifungal therapy is *not* recommended. Consider the following risk factors for candidemia: • Immunosuppression or neutropenia • Recent broad spectrum therapy • Colonization in multiple anatomic sites
Vasoactive Therapy	**Norepinephrine is preferred initial therapy** • Titrate to response until goal MAP is achieved Phenylephrine • Not recommended (see comments) Epinephrine May be added to norepinephrine or in place of (see comments) Vasopressin • May be added to norepinephrine • Up to 0.03 **unit/min**; do not titrate (doses >0.03–0.04 unit/min are for salvage)	<u>Goals:</u> Raise MAP above 65 mmHg (or SBP above 90 mmHg); central line recommended Dose ranges vary based on clinical situation Consider phenylephrine in patients w/serious arrhythmias from norepinephrine, or if cardiac output is high and blood pressure persistently low, or salvage therapy when combination of inotrope/vasopressor and low-dose vasopressin failed to achieve target MAP
Central Venous Oxygen Therapy	• If $ScvO_2$ is <70% after adequate fluid resuscitation and treatment of hypotension with persistent hypoperfusion, then dobutamine (to a maximum of 20 mcg/kg/min) or transfuse PRBC • Repeat Hgb/Hct 2 hours after transfusion • Repeat $ScvO_2$ after above intervention	<u>Goals:</u> To maintain $(ScvO_2)$ at about 70% Consider mechanical ventilation if less than 70%
Other Considerations	• Consider initiation of hydrocortisone 200 mg/day in divided doses if blood pressure is poorly responsive to IV fluids and vasoactive therapy • DVT prophylaxis for all patients • GI prophylaxis (H2 receptor antagonist proton pump inhibitor)	
Surviving Sepsis Campaign 3-hour Bundle	The following should be completed within 3 hours of severe sepsis/septic shock diagnosis: 1. Measure lactate level 2. Obtain blood cultures prior to antimicrobial administration 3. Administer broad spectrum antimicrobials 4. If septic shock, administer 30 mL/kg crystalloid for hypotension or lactate ≥4 mmol/L	Do **NOT** delay the administration of antimicrobials if blood cultures cannot be obtained

	Sepsis and Septic Shock	Comments
Surviving Sepsis Campaign 6-hour Bundle	The following should be completed within 6 hours of severe sepsis/septic shock diagnosis: 1. Repeat lactate if initial lactate was elevated 2. If hypotension persists after fluid administration: • Initiate vasopressors (for hypotension not responsive to initial fluid resuscitation) to maintain a MAP ≥65 mmHg • Repeat volume status and tissue perfusion assessment consisting of either below: **FOCUSED EXAM** *All of the following:* • Vital signs • Cardiopulmonary exam • Capillary refill evaluation • Peripheral pulse evaluation • Skin examination or *Any **two** of the following:* • Central venous pressure • Central venous oxygen measurement • Bedside cardiovascular ultrasound • Passive leg raise or fluid challenge	
Duration of Therapy	Typically 7–10 days, however, dictated by source of infection and presence or absence of bacteremia	Antimicrobials should be reassessed daily and empiric combination therapy should not continue for more than 3–5 days Empiric therapy may be de-escalated based on: • Availability of culture data • Type of isolated pathogen(s) • Patient characteristics and infection type • Preferred hospital regimens

	Sepsis and Septic Shock	Comments
Duration of Therapy		May consider the use of biomarkers especially when culture data are unavailable (e.g., procalcitonin)
		PCT can be helpful for aiding in the diagnosis, risk stratification, and monitoring sepsis. It is especially useful when the etiology is unknown to assess response to antimicrobials
		Antimicrobials should be discontinued if a noninfectious source of inflammation has been identified
		Longer duration may be needed depending on the identified pathogen (e.g., *S. aureus* bacteremia, Pseudomonal pneumonia, fungal infections, etc.)

REFERENCE

Dellinger RP, Levy MM, Rhodes A, et al. Surviving sepsis campaign: International guidelines for management of severe sepsis and septic shock: 2012. *Crit Care Med.* 2013;41:580–637.

II.13 SKIN AND SOFT TISSUE INFECTIONS AND OSTEOMYELITIS

Skin and Soft Tissue Infections (SSTI) and Osteomyelitis		Comments
Definitions	**Nonpurulent SSTIs** • **Cellulitis:** infection of the skin that may affect the dermis and epidermis and may spread to the superficial fascia • **Erysipelas:** infection of superficial skin layers and cutaneous lymphatics • **Necrotizing fasciitis:** Rare, sometimes fatal infection of the subcutaneous tissue that results in escalating destruction of the superficial fascia and subcutaneous fat	Erysipelas more common in older adults; typically on face or lower extremities
	Purulent SSTIs • **Folliculitis, furuncles, Carbuncles:** inflammation/ infection of the hair follicle • **Impetigo:** contagious superficial skin infection	Impetigo most commonly seen in children; highly contagious
	Bite Wounds • **Animal Bites:** infection from bite wounds of animals • **Human Bites:** infection from bite wounds of humans	About 90% of cat bites and/or scratches become infected com- pared to only 5–10% of dog bites
	Miscellaneous • **Diabetic Foot Infections:** infection of the foot in sites of minor penetrating trauma or nail or web space in diabetic patients • **Osteomyelitis:** infection of the bone	
Clinical Presenta- tion	**Nonpurulent SSTIs** • **Cellulitis:** redness, warm to the touch; may be accompanied by systemic symptoms (altered mental status, hypotension, fever, chills); poorly defined margins • **Erysipelas:** intense redness and painful plaque with demarcated edges typically accompanied with fever • **Necrotizing fasciitis:** greater systemic toxicity versus cellulitis; painful, shiny, tender areas with bullae; rapidly progresses	
	Purulent SSTIs • **Carbuncles:** swollen follicular mass accompanied with fever and chills • **Folliculitis:** pruritic, erythema surrounding hair follicle • **Furuncles:** erythematous nodule surrounding hair follicle that is painful • **Impetigo:** nonbullous or bullous pus-filled blisters that form a golden crust	

Skin and Soft Tissue Infections (SSTI) and Osteomyelitis		Comments
Clinical Presentation	**Bite Wounds** • **Animal Bites:** painful; discharge may be seen—infection spreads from initial point of contact • **Human Bites:** painful, throbbing extremity that is swollen with purulent discharge; range of motion decreased **Miscellaneous** • **Diabetic Foot Infections:** may see low grade fever; signs of infection may not be apparent if angiopathy or neuropathy is severe • **Osteomyelitis:** localized pain and tenderness, inflammation and decreased range of motion; may have systemic fever, chills, malaise	**Diabetic foot infections:** if infection has a foul-smelling odor, most likely anaerobes are present
Common Offending Pathogens	**Common pathogens in SSTIs:** • Gram-positive: *S. aureus, S. pyogenes* (group A strep) • Community-associated methicillin-resistant *Staphylococcus aureus* (CA-MRSA) increasing • Gram-negative: *Pseudomonas aeruginosa, E. coli*	Nonpurulent SSTIs are more commonly associated with *Streptococcus* spp. Purulent SSTIs are more commonly associated with *S. aureus* Erysipelas, impetigo, cellulitis, necrotizing fasciitis are typically considered mono-microbial Diabetic foot infections and bite wounds are typically polymicrobial

Common Offending Pathogens by SSTI	**Nonpurulent SSTIs**
	• **Cellulitis:** Group A strep and *S. aureus* (including CA-MRSA)
	• **Erysipelas:** Group A streptococcus (*S. pyogenes)* or *S. aureus*
	• **Necrotizing fasciitis Type I** (trauma and surgery)
	  ○ Anaerobes (*Bacteroides* spp., *Clostridium* spp., *Peptostreptococcus*) and facultative bacteria (*Streptococcus* spp., *Enterobacteriaceae*)
	• **Necrotizing fasciitis Type II** (streptococcal gangrene/"flesh eating bacteria")
	  ○ *S. pyogenes*	

Skin and Soft Tissue Infections (SSTI) and Osteomyelitis		Comments

Common Offending Pathogens by SSTI	**Purulent SSTIs**
	• **Carbuncles, folliculitis, furuncles:** *S. aureus* (including CA-MRSA), *P. aeruginosa* (often associated with whirlpools and hot tubs)
	• **Impetigo:** *S. aureus* and group A strep
	
	Bite Wounds
	• **Animal Bites:** Dogs and Cats: polymicrobial (*Pasturella multocida, Streptococcus* spp., *Staphylococcus* spp., *Moraxella* spp., *Neisseria* spp., *Capnocytophagia,* and anaerobes)
	• **Human Bites:** Oral flora: polymicrobial (*Eikenella corrodens, Streptococcus* spp., *S. aureus, Corynebacterium* spp., anaerobes)
	
	Miscellaneous
	• **Diabetic Foot Infections:** Mild to moderate infections are typically caused by aerobic Gram positive cocci; severe infections may be polymicrobial (*S. aureus, Streptococcus* spp., *E. coli, P. aeruginosa, Bacteroides fragilis, Peptostreptococcus*)
	• **Hematogenous Osteomyelitis**:
	  ○ *S. aureus* including MRSA
	  ○ Neonates: *S. aureus,* group B strep, *E. coli*
	  ○ Vertebral (elderly): *S. aureus, E. coli, M. tuberculosis*
	  ○ IV drug abusers: MRSA/MSSA, *P. aeruginosa*
	  ○ Sickle cell anemia: *Salmonella*
	• **Contiguous Osteomyelitis**:
	  ○ *S. aureus, P. aeruginosa, Streptococcus* spp., *E. coli, S. epidermidis*	

Empiric Treatment of Choice	**Nonpurulent SSTIs**
	• **Cellulitis:**
	  ○ Penicillinase-resistant PCN or first-generation cephalosporin typically chosen
	  ○ *Mild infection (PO therapy)*
	    ▪ Dicloxacillin 500 mg Q6h
	    ▪ Cephalexin 500 mg Q6h
	    ▪ Clindamycin 300–450 mg Q6–8h (can use if PCN allergy)
	    ▪ Penicillin V K 500 mg Q6h
	  ○ *Moderate (IV therapy)*
	    ▪ Penicillin
	    ▪ Cefazolin 1–2 g Q8h
	    ▪ Clindamycin 600–900 mg Q8h
	    ▪ Ceftriaxone 1–2g Q24h
		For nonpurulent and purulent SSTIs, treatment depends on severity of infection
		• *Mild:* no systemic signs and symptoms of infection
		• *Moderate:* systemic signs and symptoms of infection such as temperature >38°C, heart rate >90 bpm, respiratory rate >24 breaths per minute, WBC >12,000 or <400 cells/mL, or immunocompromised patients

Skin and Soft Tissue Infections (SSTI) and Osteomyelitis	Comments
Empiric Treatment of Choice	○ *Severe (IV therapy)* ▪ Surgical assessment to determine if necrotizing process ▪ Vancomycin 15–20 mg/kg Q8–24h dependent on renal function plus piperacillin/tazobactam 3.375 g Q8h (extended infusion)	• *Severe:* patients who have failed incision and drainage (I&D) plus oral anti-microbials or those with systemic signs and symptoms of infection, or immuno-compromised, or deeper infection, or organ dysfunction
	• **Erysipelas:** ○ PCN is treatment of choice and IV versus PO will depend on severity ○ *Mild-to-moderate:* ▪ IM procaine penicillin G 600,000 units Q12h or penicillin VK 250–500 mg Q6h ▪ PCN allergic: clindamycin 150–300 mg PO Q6–8h ○ *Severe:* ▪ Penicillin G 1–2 million units IV Q4–6h	For folliculitis, carbuncles, furuncles: if local heat and topical therapy ineffective after a few days, administer PO antibiotics Penicillin covers group A strep but NOT *S. aureus*—need to use a penicillinase-resistant penicillin (i.e., dicloxacillin)
	• **Necrotizing fasciitis:** ○ Empiric: Vancomycin 15–20 mg/kg IV Q8–24h depending on renal function plus piperacillin/tazobactam 3.375 g IV Q8h (extended infusion) ○ **If PCN allergic:** Vancomycin 15–20 mg/kg IV Q8–24h depending on renal function plus meropenem 2 g Q8h ○ Definitive: ▪ *S. pyogenes:* penicillin plus clindamycin ▪ *Clostridium* spp.: penicillin plus clindamycin ▪ *Aeromonas hydrophila:* doxycycline plus ciprofloxacin ▪ *Vibrio vulnificus:* doxycycline plus ceftazidime ▪ Polymicrobial: Vancomycin 15–20 mg/kg IV Q8–24h depending on renal function plus piperacillin/tazobactam 3.375 g IV Q8h (extended infusion)	TMP-SMX covers *S. aureus* but is NOT usually effective against group A strep Oral agents that may provide coverage against CA-MRSA (clindamycin, TMP-SMX, doxycycline, linezolid)

Skin and Soft Tissue Infections (SSTI) and Osteomyelitis		Comments

Empiric Treatment of Choice	**Purulent SSTIs**
	• **Carbuncles and furuncles**
	  ○ Mild (see comments for description): I&D alone
	    ▪ NO antimicrobials necessary after successful I&D
	  ○ Moderate (see comments for description): I&D (send specimen for culture and sensitivity) plus empiric sulfamethoxazole/trimethoprim (1–2 double strength tablets PO Q12h) or doxycycline (100 mg PO Q12h)
	    ▪ Definitive therapy
	      • MRSA: sulfamethoxazole/trimethoprim (1–2 double strength tablets PO Q12h)
	      • MSSA: dicloxacillin (250–500 mg PO Q6h) or cephalexin (500 mg PO Q6h)
	  ○ Severe (see comments for description): I&D (send specimen for culture and sensitivity) plus empiric vancomycin (15 mg/kg Q8–24h depending on renal function), daptomycin (4–6 mg/kg Q24h), linezolid (600 mg Q12h), telavancin (10 mg/kg Q24h), or ceftaroline (600 mg Q12h)
	    ▪ Definitive therapy
	      • MRSA: Any one of the empiric choices or sulfamethoxazole/trimethoprim if susceptible
	      • MSSA: nafcillin (1–2 g Q6h), cefazolin (1–2 g Q8h), or clindamycin (600–900 mg Q8h)
	
	• **Folliculitis**: moist heat to facilitate drainage, topical therapy (clindamycin, erythromycin, mupirocin, benzoyl peroxide) or if extensive, short course of antimicrobial therapy (same recommendations as purulent SSTIs above)
	
	• **Impetigo:**
	  ○ Dicloxacillin 250–500 mg PO Q6h
	  ○ Cephalexin 250–500 mg PO Q6h
	  ○ Cefadroxil 500 mg PO Q12h
	  ○ Clindamycin 150–300 mg PO Q6–8h
	  ○ Mupirocin ointment TOP BID (best topical agent)
	  ○ Retapamulin ointment TOP BID	

Skin and Soft Tissue Infections (SSTI) and Osteomyelitis		Comments

Empiric Treatment of Choice	**Bite Wounds**
	• **Animal Bites:**
	  ○ Oral therapy
	    ▪ Amoxicillin–clavulanate 875/125 mg BID (DOC)
	    ▪ Cefuroxime 500 mg Q12h or doxycycline 100 mg Q12h or clindamycin 300–450 mg Q8h plus FQ or clindamycin plus TMP/SMX
	    ▪ Avoid cephalexin, dicloxacillin, and erythromycin due to lack of activity against *P. multocida*
	  ○ Parenteral therapy
	    ▪ Ampicillin–sulbactam 1.5–3 g Q6-8h
	    ▪ Ciprofloxacin 400 mg Q12h plus clindamycin 600–900 Q8h
	  ○ **If PCN allergic:**
	    ▪ Ciprofloxacin 750 mg Q12h or doxycycline 100 mg Q12h PLUS clindamycin 300–450 mg Q8h
	
	• **Human Bites:**
	  ○ Oral therapy
	    ▪ Amoxicillin–clavulanate 875/125 mg BID (DOC)
	    ▪ Clindamycin 300–450 mg Q8h plus ciprofloxacin 500–750 mg Q12h
	    ▪ Clindamycin 300–450 mg Q8h plus TMP/SMX DS 1 tab Q12h
	    ▪ Avoid cephalexin, dicloxacillin, and erythromycin due to lack of activity against *Eikenella* species
	  ○ Parenteral therapy
	    ▪ Ampicillin–sulbactam 1.5–3 g Q6-8h
	    ▪ Severe: consider piperacillin–tazobactam 3.375 g Q6-8h
	    ▪ PCN allergy: clindamycin 600–900 mg Q8h plus ciprofloxacin 400 mg Q12h
	    ▪ Clindamycin 600–900 mg Q8h plus TMP/SMX
	
	Miscellaneous
	• **Diabetic Foot Infections:**
	  ○ *Mild to moderate* (typically treat with PO antimicrobials)
	  ○ Regimens with activity against *Streptococcus* spp. and MSSA
	    ▪ Dicloxacillin 500 mg Q6h (narrow spectrum, inexpensive, frequent dosing)
	    ▪ Amoxicillin/clavulanate 875/125 mg BID (broad spectrum including anaerobes)
			Do not treat uninfected wounds with antimicrobial therapy
			Mild: local infection of the skin and subcutaneous tissue, erythema >0.5 cm to ≤2 cm around ulcer with exclusion of other causes of inflammation

Skin and Soft Tissue Infections (SSTI) and Osteomyelitis		Comments

Empiric Treatment of Choice	▪ Clindamycin 300–450 mg Q6–8h (increasing rates of CA-MRSA resistance)
	▪ Cephalexin 500 mg Q6h (narrow spectrum, inexpensive, frequent dosing)
	○ Regimens with activity against CA-MRSA
	  ▪ Doxycycline 100 mg BID (relatively inexpensive, also covers some Gram negatives, variable activity against *Streptococcus* spp.)
	  ▪ TMP/SMX 1–2 DS tabs Q12h (relatively inexpensive, also covers some Gram negatives, variable activity against *Streptococcus* spp.)
	○ *Moderate-Severe* (typically initiate IV antimicrobials)
	○ Regimens with activity against streptococci, staphylococci (MSSA), *Enterobacteriaceae* and obligate anaerobes
	  ▪ Levofloxacin 750 mg Q24h (convenient dosing, inadequate *S. aureus* activity) or moxifloxacin 400 mg Q24h (convenient dosing, broad spectrum including anaerobes but excluding *Pseudomonas*)
	  ▪ Cefoxitin 1–2 g Q6–8h (frequent dosing, has anaerobic coverage)
	  ▪ Ceftriaxone 1–2 g Q24h (convenient dosing, no anaerobic or pseudomonal coverage)
		Moderate: local infection with erythema >2 cm or involving structures deeper than skin and subcutaneous tissues and no systemic inflammatory response signs
		Severe: local infection with systemic signs of infection (≥2 SIRS criteria)
		Empiric therapy targeting aerobic Gram positive cocci is reasonable in patients with mild to moderate diabetic foot infections with no recent antimicrobial exposure
		For severe diabetic foot infections, empiric therapy should be broad
		Empiric anti-pseudomonal therapy is unnecessary except for patients with risk factors (e.g., residence in a warm climate, high local prevalence, or patient with recent history of pseudomonal infection)
		Consider anti-MRSA therapy in patients with a history of MRSA infection or if local prevalence is high
		Wound care is an essential component of diabetic foot infection therapy

Skin and Soft Tissue Infections (SSTI) and Osteomyelitis	Comments

Empiric Treatment of Choice	▪ Ampicillin–sulbactam 3 g Q6h (frequent dosing, does not cover *Pseudomonas* and has high rates of *E. coli* resistance)
	▪ Ertapenem 1 g Q24h (convenient dosing, broad spectrum including anaerobes but excluding *Pseudomonas*)
	▪ Tigecycline 100 mg load, then 50 mg Q12h (broad spectrum including MRSA and anaerobes excluding *Pseudomonas*, high rates of GI adverse effects)
	▪ Meropenem 1 g Q8h or imipenem/cilastatin 500 mg Q6h (use only when required; extended-spectrum β lactamase [ESBL]–producing pathogens expected)
	◦ Regimens with activity against MRSA
	  ▪ Linezolid 600 mg Q12h
	  ▪ Daptomycin 4–6 mg/kg Q24h
	  ▪ Vancomycin 15–20 mg/kg Q12h
	◦ Regimen with activity against *Pseudomonas*
	  ▪ Piperacillin/tazobactam 3.375 g Q6h
	  ▪ Imipenem/cilastatin or meropenem
	◦ **If PCN allergic:**
	  ▪ Ciprofloxacin 750 mg Q12h or PLUS metronidazole or clindamycin
	
	• **Osteomyelitis:**
	◦ Regimens that cover MSSA
	  ▪ Nafcillin 1–2 g IV Q4–6h
	  ▪ Oxacillin 1–2 g IV Q4–6h
	  ▪ Cefazolin 1–2 g IV Q8h
	◦ Regimens that cover MRSA
	  ▪ Daptomycin 6 mg/kg IV Q 24h
	  ▪ Vancomycin 15–20 mg/kg IV Q8–24h depending on renal function
	◦ Regimens for IV drug abusers or suspect *P. aeruginosa*
	  ▪ Ceftazidime 2 g IV Q8h
	  ▪ Cefepime 2 g IV Q12h
	  ▪ Piperacillin/tazobactam 3.375 g IV Q8h (extended infusion)
	  ▪ Ciprofloxacin 400 mg IV Q8–12h
	◦ Regimens for gram positive and negative infection (post op or trauma)
	  ▪ Ceftazidime 2 g IV Q8h or
	  ▪ Piperacillin/tazobactam 3.375 g IV Q8h (extended infusion) or
	  ▪ Ciprofloxacin 400 mg IV Q8–12h PLUS	

Skin and Soft Tissue Infections (SSTI) and Osteomyelitis		Comments

Empiric Treatment of Choice	▪ Daptomycin 6 mg/kg IV Q24h or
	▪ Vancomycin 15–20 mg/kg IV Q8–24h depending on renal function
	○ Regimens that cover anaerobes
	  ▪ Clindamycin 600–900 mg IV Q8h or
	  ▪ Metronidazole 500 mg IV Q8h
	
	If β-lactam allergic:
	• Clindamycin or vancomycin	

Duration of Therapy	**Nonpurulent SSTIs** • **Cellulitis:** 5–7 days • **Erysipelas:** 7 days • **Necrotizing fasciitis:** 10–14 days; may be extended based on severity **Purulent SSTIs** • **Carbuncles:** 5–7 days • **Folliculitis:** 5–7 days • **Furuncles:** 5–7 days • **Impetigo:** 7 days **Bite Wounds** • **Animal Bites:** Non-infected (prophylaxis): 3–5 days; infected: 7–14 days • **Human Bites:** Non-infected (prophylaxis): 3–5 days; infected: 7–14 days **Miscellaneous** • **Diabetic Foot Infections:** mild-to-moderate: 1–2 weeks; severe: 2–4 weeks • **Osteomyelitis:** 4–6 weeks minimum; may be extended based on response, severity of infection, etc.	

REFERENCES

Lipsky BA, Berendt AR, Cornia PB, et al. 2012 Infectious Diseases Society of America Clinical practice guideline for the diagnosis and treatment of diabetic foot infections. *Clin Infect Dis.* 2012;54: e132–e173.

Liu C, Bayer A, Cosgrove SE, et al. Clinical practice guidelines by the Infectious Diseases Society of America for the treatment of methicillin-resistant *Staphylococcus aureus* infections in adults and children. *Clin Inf Dis.* 2011;52:1–38.

Stevens DL, Bisno AL, Chambers HF, et al. Practice guidelines for the diagnosis and management of skin and soft-tissue infections: 2014 update by the Infectious Diseases Society of America. *Clin Infect Dis.* 2012; 59(2):147–159.

II.14   URINARY TRACT INFECTIONS AND PROSTATITIS

Urinary Tract Infections (UTIs) and Prostatitis		Comments

Definition	**Acute Uncomplicated UTI:** infection in healthy females with no structural genitourinary (GU) abnormalities
	Asymptomatic Bacteriuria: presence of bacteria in urine obtained from patient with no signs or symptoms of UTI
	Bacteriuria: $\geq 10^5$ bacteria/mL (cfu/mL)
	Catheter-Associated UTI: infection caused by urinary catheterization
	Complicated UTI: infection of bladder or kidneys in patients with structural GU abnormalities
	Cystitis: inflammation/infection of bladder (lower urinary tract)
	Prostatitis: inflammation of the prostate
	Pyelonephritis: inflammation/infection of ureters and/or kidneys (upper urinary tract)
	Recurrent UTI: ≥ 2 in 6 months or ≥ 3 UTIs in a year
	• **Reinfection:** >2 weeks from initial UTI
	• **Relapse:** <2 weeks from initial UTI with same organism
	Urethritis: inflammation/infection of urethra
	Urosepsis: sepsis caused by infection of the urinary tract and/or prostate
		• UTIs confined to bladder also referred to as *lower tract infections*
		• UTIs involving the kidneys also referred to as *upper tract infections*
		• UTIs in males considered complicated UTIs
		• Asymptomatic bacteriuria is one of the most common misuses of antimicrobial therapy. Always assess patient for sign and symptoms of infection and only treat if symptoms are present regardless of CFU counts and identified pathogen.
		• Do not treat asymptomatic bacteriuria unless the patient is:
		  ○ Pregnant
		  ○ Undergoing a urologic surgical procedure

Clinical Presentation/Labs	**Laboratory Tests:**
	Positive urinalysis
	• Bacteriuria
	  ○ Any growth on suprapubic catheterization in a symptomatic patient
	  ○ $\geq 10^3$ CFU bacteria/mL in a symptomatic or catheterized patient
	  ○ $\geq 10^5$ CFU bacteria/mL in an asymptomatic patient
	• Leukocyte esterase (+): indicates white blood cells in urine
	• Nitrate (+): indicates bacteria in urine
	• Pyuria: WBC count >10/mm³
	
	Positive urine culture
		• **Lower urinary tract symptoms:** dysuria, frequency, urgency, suprapubic tenderness
		• **Upper urinary tract symptoms:** flank pain/tenderness (also referred to as CVA [costovertebral angle] tenderness), fever, nausea/vomiting
		• **Catheter-associated urinary tract symptoms:** fatigue, chills, confusion, suprapubic tenderness, CVA tenderness, fever, nausea/vomiting (dysuria, frequency, and urgency usually not present due to catheter)

Urinary Tract Infections (UTIs) and Prostatitis		Comments
Clinical Presentation/Labs		• Elderly may present with mental status changes in place of the above or may see profound weakness, frequent falls or changes in eating habits/ gastrointestinal (GI) symptoms • Concomitant interpretation of urinalysis and urine culture required in context of symptoms ○ (–) UA and (+) urine culture: likely contamination
Common Offending Pathogens	**Gram +:** • *Staphylococcus saprophyticus*	• *S. epidermidis* is common skin flora and should be considered contaminant • *Enterococcus* spp. typically seen in healthcare settings or complicated UTIs
	Gram –: • *Enterobacter* spp. • *Escherichia coli** • *Klebsiella* spp. • *Proteus mirabilis* • *Pseudomonas aeruginosa*	• **E. coli* is the most common organism to cause acute uncomplicated UTIs • *Proteus mirabilis* is most common organism isolated in men (can see alkaline urine with *Proteus* spp.)

	Empiric Treatment	Comments
Uncom-plicated Bacterial Cystitis	• TMP/SMX (avoid if local resistance >20%) • Cephalosporins (e.g., cephalexin, cefpodoxime, cefdinir) • Fluoroquinolones (e.g., ciprofloxacin, levofloxacin) • Nitrofurantoin	• Therapy commonly empiric; no culture taken • 3-day therapy preferred (5-day for nitrofurantoin) • Avoid TMP/SMX use if local resistance >20% • Fluoroquinolones typically second-line due to resistance (avoid use if local resistance >20%) • Avoid nitrofurantoin in patients with CrCl <50 ml/min • Oral fosfomycin is indicated for uncomplicated cystitis; however, due to its broad-spectrum coverage, consider reserving use for MDRO
Complicated Bacterial Cystitis	• TMP/SMX • Cephalosporins (e.g., cephalexin, cefpodoxime, cefdinir) • Fluoroquinolones (e.g., ciprofloxacin, levofloxacin) • Nitrofurantoin	• 7–14 day treatment course • Avoid TMP/SMX use if local resistance >20% • Avoid fluoroquinolone use if local resistance >20% • Avoid nitrofurantoin in patients with CrCl <50 ml/min • Oral fosfomycin × 2–3 doses separated by 48–72 hours (broad-spectrum coverage; consider reserving use for MDRO)
Pyelo-nephritis	<u>IV</u> • Extended-spectrum cephalosporin (e.g., ceftriaxone, cefepime) • Ertapenem <u>PO</u> • Fluoroquinolones (e.g., ciprofloxacin, levofloxacin) • TMP/SMX • Cefpodoxime	• Typical presentation for mild-moderate pyelonephritis: low-grade temperature, stable vital signs • Typical presentation for severe pyelonephritis: fever <100.9°F, vomiting, dehydration, signs of sepsis

	Empiric Treatment	Comments
Pyelo-nephritis		• Hospitalization/initial therapy with IV antibiotics • If multiple PCN and cephalosporin allergies: aztreonam • Avoid TMP/SMX use if local resistance >20% • 7–14 day treatment course
Urinary Tract Infections in Men	• Fluoroquinolones • TMP/SMX	• Nitrofurantoin and β-lactams not typically used due to inadequate tissue concentrations • Avoid TMP/SMX use if local resistance >20% • If young male, can consider 7-day course • 7–14 day treatment course
Catheter-Associated Urinary Tract Infections	• Ertapenem • Extended-spectrum cephalosporin (e.g., ceftriaxone, cefepime) • Fluoroquinolones	When to change catheters? • If catheter has been in place >2 weeks and is still indicated, change catheter. Urine culture should be obtained after new catheter is placed and before antimicrobial therapy is initiated. Duration of Treatment • If prompt resolution of symptoms: 7 days • If delayed response: 7–14 days • Women <65 years with without upper urinary tract symptoms after an indwelling catheter has been removed: 3 days
Urinary Tract Infections in Pregnancy	• Amoxicillin/clavulanate • Cephalosporin • Nitrofurantoin • Fosfomycin	• Screened at baseline and 28 weeks • 7-day treatment course (exception fosfomycin: single dose) • Fosfomycin has broad-spectrum coverage; consider reserving use for MDRO

	Empiric Treatment	Comments
Urinary Tract Infections in Pregnancy		• **AVOID:** ✓ Tetracyclines ✓ Fluoroquinolones ✓ TMP/SMX in third trimester • Follow-up culture and monthly cultures thereafter recommended
Prostatitis	• Fluoroquinolones (preferred) • TMP/SMX	• Prolonged treatment necessary to reach colonies of bacteria deep within prostate gland • Avoid TMP/SMX use if local resistance >20% • 4–6 week treatment course
Urosepsis	• Extended-spectrum cephalosporin (e.g., ceftriaxone, cefepime) • Fluoroquinolones	• Oral β-lactams not effective due to inadequate blood concentrations • If multiple PCN and cephalosporin allergies: aztreonam • 7–14 day treatment course
Enterococci	*E. faecalis* • Ampicillin • Amoxicillin *E. faecium* • Nitrofurantoin • Fosfomycin • Linezolid • Vancomycin (if susceptible)	• In PCN allergy: nitrofurantoin • *E. faecium* often resistant to vancomycin • 5–7 day treatment course (Exception for fosfomycin: single-dose therapy for uncomplicated enterococcal UTI or 2–3 doses for complicated enterococcal UTI)
Prevention of Recurrent Infection	Self-administered prophylaxis • Post-coital prophylaxis ✓ TMP/SMX x 1 dose • Low-dose prophylaxis ✓ TMP/SMX ✓ Fluoroquinolones ✓ Nitrofurantoin • Post-menopausal females ✓ Topical estrogen therapy	• If initiated, after 4–6 months of prophylaxis, it is important to reassess and determine continued need with a trial off of prophylactic antimicrobial

	Empiric Treatment	Comments

Prevention of Recurrent Infection		• If recurrent infection is considered a relapse:
		  ✓ Options listed under self-administered prophylaxis prescribed as a 14-day treatment course
		  ✓ Urologic examination is advised
		  ✓ Commonly indicates prostatitis in male patients

Additional Comments	• Amoxicillin or ampicillin should not be used for empiric treatment ✓ Exception: treatment of *Enterococcus* in the urine • Do not use moxifloxacin due to insufficient urinary concentration • Follow-up cultures are not necessary for cystitis or pyelonephritis that has responded adequately to antimicrobials • Resistance to TMP/SMX and fluoroquinolones is increasing • *Candida* spp. are a common colonizer in critically ill and catheterized patients; rarely warrants antifungal therapy unless the patient has concomitant candidemia or signs/symptoms of infection without another identified source	

REFERENCES

Gupta K, Hooton TM, Naber KG, et al. International clinical practice guidelines for the treatment of acute uncomplicated cystitis and pyelonephritis in women: a 2010 update by the Infectious Diseases Society of America and the European Society for Microbiology and Infectious Diseases. *Clin Infect Dis.* 2011;52(5):e103–e120.

Hooton TM, Bradley SF, Cardenas DD, et al. Diagnosis, prevention, and treatment of catheter-associated urinary tract infection in adults: 2009 international clinical practice guidelines from the Infectious Diseases Society of America. *Clin Infect Dis.* 2010;50:625–663.

Nicolle LE, Bradley SF, Colgan R, et al. Infectious Diseases Society of America guidelines for the diagnosis and treatment of asymptomatic bacteriuria in adults. *Clin Infect Dis.* 2005;40:643–654.

❖ ❖ ❖

PART III

What Anti-Infectives Provide Adequate Coverage for the Suspected Infection?

III.1 ANTIFUNGALS

III.2 ANTIMICROBIALS

III.3 ANTIVIRALS

III.1.1   AZOLES

Antifungal	Ketoconazole	Fluconazole	Isavuconazole	Itraconazole	Miconazole/ Clotrimazole	Voriconazole	Posaconazole
Mechanism of Action	Inhibits 14-alpha-demethylation of lanosterol, thereby reducing ergosterol synthesis resulting in increased cell permeability and leakage of essential cell components						
Spectrum of Activity	Treats fungal infections						
FDA-Approved Indications	Blastomycosis Candidiasis (vulvovaginitis, cutaneous, mucocutaneous, esophagitis) Candiduria Chromoblastomycosis Coccidioidomycosis Histoplasmosis Paracoccidioidomycosis Severe recalcitrant tinea infections (corporis, cruris, pedis)	Candidiasis (prophylaxis, vulvovaginitis, candidemia, esophagitis, candiduria, oropharyngeal) Cryptococcal meningitis, treatment and suppression	Invasive Aspergillosis Invasive Mucormycosis	Aspergillosis (salvage) Blastomycosis Candidiasis (esophageal, oropharyngeal) Histoplamosis Onchomycosis	Oropharyngeal candidiasis Candidal vulvovaginitis	Aspergillosis Candidemia Candidiasis (esophageal; disseminated; involving the abdomen, skin, kidney, bladder, and wounds) Scedosporium apiospermum Fusarium spp.	Aspergillosis prophylaxis Disseminated candidiasis, prophylaxis Oropharyngeal candidiasis

Non-FDA-Approved Indications	Allescheriosis Atopic dermatitis Prostate carcinoma Neonatal candidiasis Diseminated candidiasis, prophylaxis	Coccidioidomycosis Histoplasmosis (itraconazole preferred) Pityriasis versicolor Endophthalmitis Candida prophylaxis in surgical patients	—	Candidal vulvovaginitis Coccidioidomycosis Cryptococcosis Paracoccidioidomycosis Penicilliosis Sporotrichosis	Tinea infections	Blastomycosis Candida endophthalmitis Candidiasis, oropharyngeal Scedosporium prolificans Empiric therapy for febrile neutropenia	Aspergillosis Esophageal candidiasis Fusarium infection Zygomycoses
Pharmacodynamics	AUC/MIC Fungistatic; unlikely to exhibit fungicidal activity as unattainable concentrations would be required; + PAE	AUC/MIC; fungistatic; + PAE	AUC/MIC; fungistatic	AUC/MIC; fungistatic	AUC/MIC; fungistatic		
Pharmacokinetics	Partially metabolized and excreted in feces	Renally eliminated (80% unchanged)	Hepatic metabolism; excreted in urine and feces	Hepatic metabolism; excreted in urine and feces	Hepatic metabolism (systemic); excretion in urine and feces	Hepatic metabolism; excretion in urine	Metabolized by glucuronidation; excreted in feces and urine

(continued)

Antifungal	Ketoconazole	Fluconazole	Isavuconazole	Itraconazole	Miconazole/Clotrimazole	Voriconazole	Posaconazole
Distribution	Bone—poor CNS—poor Fluids—readily Tissues—readily	CNS—readily Fluids—readily Tissues—readily	Fluids—readily Tissues—readily	CNS—negligible Fluids—readily Tissues—readily	CNS—poor Tissues—readily	CNS—readily Fluids—readily Tissues—readily	Widely distributed
Adverse Effects	Asthenia Elevated LFTs GI Headache, dizziness Hepatitis	Alopecia (long-term use; doses >400 mg daily) Anorexia GI Headache QT prolongation Seizures (high doses) Torsades de pointes (rare) Usually well tolerated	Peripheral edema HA Hypokalemia GI Elevated LFTs Infusion-related reactions (hypotension, chills, dyspnea, dizziness, paresthesia)	Adrenal insufficiency (long-term high-dose use) Cardiotoxicity (negative inotropic effect) Elevated LFTs GI Gynecomastia Headache Neuropathy Rash	Pruritis Contact dermatitis Rash Altered taste/GI (oral)	Visual disturbances (blurriness, color changes, and enhanced vision) in ~21% of patients; duration usually lasts <30 minutes and occurs typically 30 minutes after dosing (most common with IV formulation) Elevated LFTs/bilirubin Rash (photosensitive) Hallucination/encephalopathy (troughs >5.5 mcg/mL) GI	Usually well tolerated Hypokalemia Headache GI Elevated LFTs/bilirubin QT prolongation

| Drug Interactions | Substrate and potent inhibitor of CYP3A4

Contraindicated:
Astemizole
Cisapride
Midazolam
Pimozide
Quinidine
Terfenadine
Triazolam

Avoid:
Proton pump inhibitors
H2 blockers
Antacid (due to pH-dependent absorption) | CYP3A4, CYP2C9, CYP2C19 substrate

Contraindicated:
Alfuzosin
Astemizole
Bepridil
Cisapride
Citalopram
Clozapine
Crizotinib
Dasatinib
Dromperidone
Dronedarone
Granisetron
Lapatinib
Levomethadyl
Lomitapide
Lumefantrine
Mesoridazine
Mifepristone
Nilotinib
Ondansetron
Pimozide
Quetiapine
Salmeterol
Sorafenib
Sparfloxacin
Sunitinib
Terfenadine | CYP3A4 substrate CYP2C19, CYP2C8, CYP2C9, CYP2D6, CYP3A4, P-glycoprotein inhibitor

CYP2B6, CYP2C8, CYP2C9, and CYP3A4 inducer

Contraindicated:
Amodiaquine
Bosutinib
Conivaptan
CYP3A4 (strong) inducers
Domperidone
Ibrutinib
Idelalisib
Ivabradine
Lomitapide
Naloxegol
Olaparib
Pimozide | CYP3A4 inhibitor

Contraindicated:
Alfuzosin
Alprazolam, Midazolam, Triazolam
Astemizole
Cisapride
Colchicine
Conivaptan
Dofetilide
Dronedarone
Eplerenone
Ergot Derivatives
Felodipine
Levomethadyl
Lomitapide
Lovastatin
Maraviroc
Methadone
Nimodipine
Nislodipine
Pimozide
Quinidine
Ranolazine
Silodosin
Simvastatin, Terfenadine
Tolvaptan | Pimozide | CYP2C19, CYP2C9, CYP3A4

Contraindicated:
Astemizole
Barbiturates
Carbamazepine
Cisapride
Dronedarone
Ergot Derivatives
Lomitapide
Lovastatin
Simvastatin
Lurasidone
Mesoridazine
Miraviroc
Nimodipine
Pimozide
Posaconazole
Primidone
Quinidine
Rifabutin
Rifampin
Ritonavir
Sirolimus
Sparfloxacin
St. John's Wort
Terfenadine
Thioridazine | Substrate P-gp efflux and CYP3A4 inhibitor

Contraindicated:
Alfuzosin
Amiodarone
Astemizole
Atorvastatin
Cisapride
Citalopram
Clarithromycin
Clozapine
Crizotinib
Dasatinib
Disopyramide
Dofetilide
Domperidone
Dronedarone
Ergot Derivatives
Erythromycin
Halofantrine
Iloperidone
Lapatinib
Lomitapide
Lopinavir
Lovastatin
Lumefantrine
Lurasidone
Maraviroc
Mefloquine |
|---|---|---|---|---|---|---|---|

(continued)

Antifungal	Ketoconazole	Fluconazole	Isavuconazole	Itraconazole	Miconazole/ Clotrimazole	Voriconazole	Posaconazole
Drug Interactions (Cont'd)		Thioridazine Vardenafil Ziprasidone	*Saccharomyces boulardii* Simeprevir St. John's Wort Tolvaptan Trabectedin Ulipristal	Avoid: Proton pump inhibitors H2 blockers Antacid (due to pH-dependent absorption)			Mesoridazine Methadone Mifepristone Nilotinib Nimodipine Ondansetron Pazopanib Pimozide Propafenone Quetiapine Quinidine Quinine Ranolizine Salmeterol Saquinavir Simvastatin Sirolimus Solifenacin Sorafenib Sparfloxacin Sunitinib Telithromycin Terfenadine Thioridazine Toremifene Trazodone Vardenafil Vemurafenib Voriconazole Ziprasidone

Dose	200–800 mg/day; dose depends on indication	Large-range 100–1,200 mg/day; dose depends on indication Patients who are obese may require larger doses Larger doses are required when isolate deemed susceptible dose dependent	IV and PO Load: 372 mg (isavuconazole 200 mg) Q8h for 6 doses; Maintenance 372 mg (isavuconazole 200 mg) once daily Start maintenance 12–24h after the last loading dose	Loading dose of 200 mg Q8h × 3 days for all serious infections 200–400 mg PO Q12h	Cream applied Q12h for tinea Vaginal: once daily or clotrimazole Q12h × 3 days Clotrimazole Troches 5X/day Miconazole Buccal once daily	6 mg/kg Q12h × 2 doses, then 4 mg/kg Q12h IV usually used to load 200–300 mg PO Q12h 6 mg/kg Q12h × 2 doses, then 2 mg/kg Q12h in hepatic insufficiency	Avoid: Proton pump inhibitors H2 blockers Antacid (due to pH-dependent absorption) Oral suspension: 200 mg PO Q8h (prophylaxis) Delayed-release tablets or IV: 300 mg Q12h on day 1 then 300 mg once daily (prophylaxis and treatment) Oral suspension: 200 mg PO Q6h or 400 mg PO Q12h (treatment)

(continued)

Antifungal	Ketoconazole	Fluconazole	Isavuconazole	Itraconazole	Miconazole/ Clotrimazole	Voriconazole	Posaconazole
Dose (Cont'd)							100 mg PO Q12h × 2 doses, then 100 mg PO Q24h for oropharyngeal candidiasis
Monitoring		Renal function	LFTs Infusion-related reactions	Target serum concentration: 1–2 mcg/mL 2 hours after dose after 5 days of therapy for treatment; >0.5 mcg/mL for prophylaxis		Target serum concentration: >1–2 mcg/mL and <6 mcg/mL within 2 hours of the next dose; prior to the third dose in patients who received load or after 7 days of therapy in patients who did not receive a load for treatment; >0.5 mcg/mL may be sufficient for prophylaxis	Potential target serum concentrations for prophylaxis and treatment of invasive aspergillosis are 0.7 mcg/mL and 1.25 mcg/mL, respectively Levels should be assessed after 1 week of therapy

							Goal trough/ MIC ratio of 2–5 is associated with the highest probability of response
	All systemic azoles: LFTs						
Resistance Mechanisms	Cross-resistance within the azole class common; Efflux pumps; Target point mutations	C. krusei, C. lusitaniae resistant, and 30–40% of C. glabrata resistant					
Comments	Absorption dependent on gastric acidity; administer with acidic drinks. Used for prostate cancer	~90% oral bioavailability; no effect of food or gastric pH	Isavuconazole sulfate is a prodrug rapidly hydrolyzed in the blood to active isavuconazole. 98% oral bioavailability	Absorption dependent on gastric acidity; administer with acidic drinks. Oral solution has superior bioavailability than capsules. Oral solution should be taken on an empty stomach	Buccal tablets; hold tablet in place and allow to dissolve. Do **NOT** crush, chew, or swallow tablets. Also available as vaginal cream/suppository and topical cream	Absorption independent on gastric acidity but reduced by 24% with high fat meals, thus PO best absorbed on an empty stomach. Evidence of treatment failure in patients who have trough concentrations <1.7 mcg/mL. Suspension well absorbed when administered with food or nutritional supplement; acidic beverage helps absorption as well. Potential saturable absorption at doses >800 mg/day	

(continued)

Antifungal	Ketoconazole	Fluconazole	Isavuconazole	Itraconazole	Miconazole/ Clotrinazole	Voriconazole	Posaconazole
Comments *(Cont'd)*		In patients with chronic, prolonged, or repeated courses of fluconazole, resistance can develop. May overcome by increasing the dose or may require an alternative antifungal		Capsules should be taken on a full stomach 200-mg capsule = 100-mg oral solution		IV formulation not recommended in CrCl <50 mL/min due to toxicity potential of the sulfobutylether-cyclodextrin vehicle No reliable activity against zygomycetes Increasing patient age may increase voriconazole levels; increased patient weight may decrease voriconazole levels	Do **NOT** use the delayed-release tablet and oral suspension interchangeably due to dosing differences for each formulation IV formulation contains cyclodextrin and may accumulate in renal insufficiency (eGFR <50 mL/min/1.73 m³); If increases in SCr occur while on IV therapy consider switch to oral

III.1.2 ECHINOCANDINS

Antifungal	Anidulafungin (IV)	Caspofungin (IV)	Micafungin (IV)
Mechanism of Action	Inhibits 1,3 beta-D-glucan synthase, the enzyme required for polysaccharide formation in the fungal cell wall		
Spectrum of Activity	Candida spp. Aspergillus spp. Candida parapsilosis may be resistant No activity against Cryptococcus neoformans, zygomycetes, Trichosporon spp., and Fusarium spp.		
FDA-Approved Indications	Candidemia and other candida infections (intra-abdominal, peritonitis) Poor CNS penetration	Invasive Aspergillosis in patients refractory or intolerant to other antifungal therapy Candidemia Esophageal candidiasis Empiric antifungal therapy, febrile neutropenia	Candidemia Esophageal candidiasis Candidiasis prophylaxis
Non-FDA-Approved Indications	Aspergillosis Endophthalmitis Empiric antifungal therapy for suspected candidiasis	Aspergillosis Endophthalmitis Invasive fungal infection prophylaxis	Aspergillosis Endophthalmitis Empiric antifungal therapy for suspected candidiasis
Pharmacodynamics	Concentration dependent (C_{max}/MIC of 10; AUC/MIC > 20); fungicidal, + PAE		
Pharmacokinetics	Metabolized by N-acetylation and hydrolysis; eliminated in the urine and feces		
Distribution	Bone—poor CSF—poor Tissues—readily Urine—poor		
Adverse Effects	Generally well-tolerated GI HA Hypersensitivity reaction (infusion rate related)		

(continued)

Antifungal	Anidulafungin (IV)	Caspofungin (IV)	Micafungin (IV)
Adverse Effects *(Cont'd)*	Hypokalemia (anidulafungin, micafungin) LFT/bilirubin elevations Phlebitis		
Drug Interactions	Cyclosporin: anidulafungin AUC ↑ 22%	Carbamazepine Cyclosporine Dexamethasone Efavirenz Etravirine Nevirapine Phenobarbital Phenytoin Rifabutin Rifampin Tacrolimus	Itraconazole Nifedipine Sirolimus
Dose	200 mg × 1 then 100 mg Q24h 100 mg × 1, then 50 mg Q24h for esophageal candidasis	70 mg IV day 1, then 50 mg Q24h Obese patients 70 mg IV Q24h Decrease maintenance dose to 35 mg IV Q24h after normal load in patients with hepatic dysfunction	100–150 mg IV Q24h 50 mg IV Q24h for prophylaxis
Monitoring	Liver Function Potassium Renal Function		
Resistance Mechanisms	Direct changes in the glucan synthase enzyme complex that affects echinocandin binding		
Comments	Echinocandins retain activity against biofilm embedded *Candida* spp. Should be reserved for azole-resistant *Candida* infections		

III.1.3   FLUCYTOSINE

Antifungal	Flucytosine
Mechanism of Action	Interferes with protein synthesis by incorporation into fungal RNA after being converted to 5-FU intracellularly
Spectrum of Activity	Treats fungal infections—*Candida* spp., *Cryptococcus* spp.
FDA-Approved Indications	Candidiasis Cryptococcal infections
Non-FDA-Approved Indications	Candida endophthalmitis CNS Candidiasis
Pharmacodynamics	T > MIC; fungistatic; + PAE
Pharmacokinetics	Renal elimination (85–95% unchanged)
Distribution	CNS—readily Fluids—readily Tissues—readily
Adverse Effects	Altered taste Bone marrow suppression CNS effects (confusion) GI Headache Hepatitis Peripheral neuropathy Photosensitivity Pruritis Rash
Drug Interactions	Cytarabine (antagonism) Other bone marrow suppressing agents
Dose	25 mg/kg PO Q6h Use ideal body weight in obese patients
Monitoring	Therapeutic drug monitoring recommended, especially in renal insufficiency Goal peak 50–100 mcg/mL 2 hours post dose at steady state
Resistance Mechanisms	Mechanisms unknown
Comments	Flucytosine should not be used as monotherapy as resistance develops quickly

III.1.4 POLYENES

Antifungal	Amphotericin B Deoxycholate	Amphotericin B-Lipid Complex (ABLC, Abelcet)	Liposomal Amphotericin B (AmBisome)	Amphotericin B Colloidal Dispersion (ABCD)	Nystatin
Mechanism of Action	Binds to ergosterol in fungal cell membrane and induces excessive permeability of the plasma membrane resulting in leakage of essential cell components with subsequent cell death				
Spectrum of Activity	Broad spectrum; treats fungal and mold infections				
FDA-Approved Indications	Aspergillosis, invasive Basidiobolus Blastomycosis Candidiasis, disseminated Coccidioidomycosis Conidiobolus Cryptococcal meningitis (treatment and suppression) Cryptococcosis Fungal infection of the CNS, lung, or urinary tract Histoplasmosis Leishmaniasis Mucormycosis Sporotrichosis	Aspergillosis, invasive Blastomycosis Leishmaniasis Systemic mycosis Candidiasis Cryptococcosis For patients who are refractory or intolerant to conventional amphotericin B	Aspergillosis, invasive Candidiasis, disseminated Cryptococcal meningitis (treatment and suppression) Cryptococcosis Empiric antifungal therapy in febrile neutropenia Leishmaniasis	Aspergillosis, invasive (for patients who are refractory or intolerant to conventional amphotericin B)	Candidiasis, cutaneous, mucocutaneous, oropharyngeal, vulvovaginal
Non-FDA-Approved Indications	Aspergillosis, invasive (+ HIV infection) Coccidioidomycosis (+ HIV infection)	Aspergillosis, invasive (+ HIV infection) Coccidioidomycosis (+/− HIV infection)	Aspergillosis, invasive (+ HIV infection) Blastomycosis	Candidiasis Leishmaniasis	—

Non-FDA-Approved Indications (*Cont'd*)	Cryptococcosis (+ HIV infection) Disseminated candidiasis (chronic or + HIV infection) Empiric antifungal therapy (febrile neutropenia or + HIV infection) Esophageal candidiasis (+/– HIV infection) Naegleria Neonatal candidiasis Oropharyngeal candidiasis Penicillium marneffei Renal tract candidiasis Suspected candidiasis in nonneutropenic patients	Cryptococcal meningitis (+ HIV infection) Cryptococcosis (+ HIV infection) Disseminated candidiasis (chronic or + HIV infection) Empiric antifungal therapy, suspected candidiasis Esophageal candidiasis (+ HIV infection) Histoplasmosis (+ HIV infection) Oropharyngeal candidiasis Sporotrichosis	Coccidioidomycosis (+/– HIV infection) Cryptococcosis (+ HIV infection) Disseminated candidiasis (chronic or solid-organ transplant recipients) Prophylaxis Disseminated candidiasis–HIV infection Esophageal candidiasis (+ HIV infection) Histoplasmosis Histoplasmosis–HIV infection HIV infection–oropharyngeal candidiasis Invasive pulmonary aspergillosis; prophylaxis Mycosis; prophylaxis Neonatal candidiasis Sporotrichosis
Pharmaco-dynamics	C_{max}/MIC and AUC/MIC; fungicidal		Unknown
Pharmaco-kinetics	Metabolism not understood; slow renal excretion		Poorly absorbed; excreted in the feces as unchanged drug

(*continued*)

Antifungal	Amphotericin B Deoxycholate	Amphotericin B-Lipid Complex (ABLC, Abelcet)	Liposomal Amphotericin B (AmBisome)	Amphotericin B Colloidal Dispersion (ABCD)	Nystatin
Distribution	CNS—poor (effective for cryptococcal meningitis) Fluids—readily Tissues—readily	Fluids—readily Increased liver, spleen uptake, however, decreased kidney uptake compared to conventional amphotericin B Lower serum concentration, higher V_d compared to conventional Tissues—readily			Saliva No systemic absorption
Adverse Effects	Anemia Bilirubin elevation GI Headache Hypocalcemia Hypokalemia Hypomagnesemia Hypotension Infusion-related reaction (fever, chills, nausea, vomiting, and rigors) • More common with deoxycholate Insomnia LFT elevation Metallic taste Nephrotoxicity Phlebitis				GI Rash (severe: Stevens-Johnson syndrome) Skin irritation
Drug Interactions	Corticosteroids (hypokalemia) Digoxin (increased incidence of digoxin toxicity due to hypokalemia) Diuretics (hypokalemia) Nephrotoxic agents (cidofovir, foscarnet, aminoglycosides, pentamidine, etc.) Skeletal muscle relaxants (enhanced effect due to hypokalemia)				None

Dose No renal dose adjustments required	0.3–1.5 mg/kg/day IV infuse over 2–4 hours Use actual body weight for obese patients	5 mg/kg/day IV Use ideal body weight for obese patients	3–5 mg/kg/day Use ideal body weight for obese patients	3–4 mg/kg/day IV or 6 mg/kg/day IV for Aspergillosis Use ideal body weight for obese patients	500,000 to 1,000,000 Units 3–5X daily 1 vaginal tablet (100,000 units) daily Topical: apply Q12h
Monitoring	Electrolytes (K, Mg, Ca) Renal function				Local reactions
Resistance	*Candida lusitaniae, Pseudallescheria boydii* are resistant Some *Fusarium oxysporum* and *F. solani* are resistant				Some *Candida* spp. Usually occurs after exposure to drug
Comments	Nephrotoxicity may be reduced with adequate hydration (500 mL 0.9% NaCl pre- and post-infusion) Infusion-related reactions common Infusion-related reactions may be immediate but usually occur within 15 minutes–4 hours post administration	Infusion-related reaction less likely; consider pre-meds if reactions develop Infusion-related reactions may be immediate but usually occur within 15 minutes–4 hours post administration	Infusion-related reaction less likely; consider pre-meds if reactions develop Infusion-related reactions may be immediate but usually occur within 15 minutes–4 hours post administration	Infusion-related actions common Infusion-related reactions may be immediate but usually occur within 15 minutes–4 hours post administration	Swish in mouth as long as possible before spitting or swallowing to allow maximum exposure Poor taste (oral)

(continued)

Antifungal	Amphotericin B Deoxycholate	Amphotericin B-Lipid Complex (ABLC, Abelcet)	Liposomal Amphotericin B (AmBisome)	Amphotericin B Colloidal Dispersion (ABCD)	Nystatin
Comments (*Cont'd*)	Symptoms may be reduced by administration of the following medications prior to infusion: Acetaminophen 650–1000 mg or Ibuprofen 200–400 mg Diphenhydramine 25–50 mg IV or PO Meperidine 25–50 mg (for chills/rigors)—avoid in renal impairment Hydrocortisone 25 mg (for Phlebitis) Prochlorperazine 10 mg or ondansetron 4 mg (GI effects) Can also cause renal tubular acidosis	Symptoms may be reduced by administration of the following medications prior to infusion: Acetaminophen 650–1000 mg or Ibuprofen 200–400 mg Diphenhydramine 25–50 mg IV or PO Meperidine 25–50 mg (for chills/rigors)—avoid in renal impairment Hydrocortisone 25 mg (for Phlebitis) Prochlorperazine 10 mg or ondansetron 4 mg (GI effects)	Symptoms may be reduced by administration of the following medications prior to infusion: Acetaminophen 650–1000 mg or Ibuprofen 200–400 mg Diphenhydramine 25–50 mg IV or PO Meperidine 25–50 mg (for chills/rigors)—avoid in renal impairment Hydrocortisone 25 mg (for Phlebitis) Prochlorperazine 10 mg or ondansetron 4 mg (GI effects) Alternative to conventional for cryptococcal meningitis	Symptoms may be reduced by administration of the following medications prior to infusion: Acetaminophen 650–1000 mg or Ibuprofen 200–400 mg Diphenhydramine 25–50 mg IV or PO Meperidine 25–50 mg (for chills/rigors)—avoid in renal impairment Hydrocortisone 25 mg (for Phlebitis) Prochlorperazine 10 mg or ondansetron 4 mg (GI effects) Other lipid formulations preferred due to highest incidence of adverse effects, especially infusion-related reaction with ABCD	

III.2 ANTIMICROBIALS

III.2.1   AMINOGLYCOSIDES

Antimicrobial	Aminoglycosides
Examples	Amikacin (IV) Gentamicin (IV, topical) Neomycin (PO, topical) Streptomycin (IV, IM) Tobramycin (IV, inhaled)
Mechanism of Action	Inhibits protein synthesis (30S subunit)
Spectrum of Activity	**Gram +:** synergistic ONLY (gentamicin) **Gram −:** includes most community and nosocomial pathogens, including *Pseudomonas* (does not cover gram (−) cocci well [*Neisseria, Moraxella, H. flu*]) **Anaerobes:** None **Atypical:** None
FDA-Approved Indications	Bacteremia Eye infections Infective endocarditis Intra-abdominal infections (in combination with agents that have gram-positive and anaerobic coverage) LRTI (poor penetration) Meningitis (poor penetration) Neonatal sepsis Osteomyelitis SSTI UTI
Non-FDA-Approved Indications	Cystic fibrosis exacerbations Neutropenic fever (adjunct) PID (in combination with clindamycin) Surgical prophylaxis Tularemia

Pharmacodynamics	C_{max}/MIC, bactericidal, + PAE
Pharmacokinetics	Renal elimination
Distribution	Body fluids—readily Placenta—crosses Tissues and bone—variable
Adverse Effects	Irreversible ototoxicity (cochlear and vestibular) Neuromuscular junction blockage Nephrotoxicity (usually reversible)
Drug Interactions	Loop diuretics (especially ethacrynic acid) due to increased cochlear toxicity Neuromuscular blocking agents—may result in enhanced and/or prolonged neuromuscular blockade, which may lead to respiratory depression and paralysis Other oto/nephrotoxic medications
Dose **Renal dose adjustments required. Refer to Amino-glycoside Dosing and Pharmacokinetics**	**Gentamicin and Tobramycin** Once daily dosing: 5–7 mg/kg; goal trough <1 mcg/mL Traditional dosing for mild-to-moderate infections: 2 mg/kg IV Q8h; goals: trough <2 mcg/mL, peak >6 mcg/mL Traditional dosing for severe infections: 3 mg/kg load then 2 mg/kg IV Q8h; goals: trough <2 mcg/mL, peak >8 mcg/mL Synergistic gentamicin dosing: 1 mg/kg Q8h; goals: trough <1 mcg/mL, peak <3–5 mcg/mL Intraventricular preservative-free gentamicin or tobramycin: 5 mg Q24h (range 4–10 mg) Nebulized tobramycin: 300 mg Q12–24h Ideal body weight should be used to calculate dose; if obese, use adjusted body weight **Amikacin** Once daily dosing: 15–20 mg/kg; goal trough <4 mcg/mL Traditional dosing for mild-to-moderate infections: 8 mg/kg load, then 7 mg/kg IV Q8h; goals: trough <10 mcg/mL, peak 20–30 mcg/mL Traditional dosing for severe infections: 8–12 mg/kg load then 8 mg/kg IV Q8h; goals: trough <10 mcg/mL, peak 25–35 mcg/mL Intraventricular amikacin (not available as preservative free; only use if pathogen is gentamicin and tobramycin resistant as sodium bisulfate may increase neurotoxicity risk): 15 mg Q24h (range 10–50 mg)

(continued)

Antimicrobial	Aminoglycosides
Monitoring	Auditory testing at baseline and follow-up determined by anticipated duration in patients receiving aminoglycosides for a prolonged duration (i.e., infective endocarditis or antipated duration ≥14 days) Renal function Serum peak and trough concentrations; trough should be drawn 30 minutes prior to the fourth dose, and peaks should be drawn 30 minutes after the end of a 30-minute infusion
Resistance Mechanisms	Alteration of ribosomal site Aminoglycoside-modifying enzymes Decreased cell permeability Efflux pumps
Comments	Aminoglycosides are generally used in combination with other antimicrobials (uncomplicated UTIs are an exception) Avoid once-daily dosing in patients with unstable renal function, endocarditis, meningitis, or in patients with an altered volume of distribution (ascites, pregnancy, burn patients) Peak affected by the dose; troughs affected by the dosing interval; peaks correlate with efficacy and potentially ototoxicity (although controversial); troughs may correlate with nephrotoxicity (especially when elevated for prolonged periods)

III.2.2 CARBAPENEMS

Antimicrobial	Ertapenem	Imipenem/Cilastatin	Meropenem	Doripenem
Mechanism of Action	Inhibits cell wall synthesis			
Spectrum of Activity	**Gram +:** *Staphylococcus* (MSSA, MSSE), *Streptococcus* excluding penicillin-resistant *S. pneumoniae*	**Gram +:** *Staphylococcus* (MSSA, MSSE), *Streptococcus* including penicillin-resistant *S. pneumoniae*, *Enterococcus faecalis* (vancomycin-susceptible only)	**Gram +:** *Staphylococcus* (MSSA, MSSE), *Streptococcus* including penicillin-resistant *S. pneumoniae*, Listeria, +/– *Enterococcus faecalis* (vancomycin-susceptible only)	**Gram +:** *Staphylococcus* (MSSA, MSSE), *Streptococcus* including penicillin-resistant *S. pneumoniae*, +/– *Enterococcus faecalis* (vancomycin-susceptible)
	Gram –: Broad—including ESBL-producing organisms; no *Pseudomonas* or *Acinetobacter* coverage	**Gram –:** Broad—including ESBL-producing organisms, *Pseudomonas*, and some *Acinetobacter* isolates	**Gram –:** Broad—including ESBL-producing organisms, *Pseudomonas*, some *Acinetobacter* isolates, *Burkholderia*	**Gram –:** Broad—including ESBL-producing organisms, *Pseudomonas*, some *Acinetobacter* isolates, *Burkholderia*
	Anaerobes: Broad—including *Bacteroides fragilis* and *Clostridium* spp. (not *C. difficile*)	**Anaerobes:** Broad—including *Bacteroides fragilis* and *Clostridium* spp. (not *C. difficile*)	**Anaerobes:** Broad—including *Bacteroides fragilis* and *Clostridium* spp. (not *C. difficile*)	**Anaerobes:** Broad—including *Bacteroides fragilis* and *Clostridium* spp. (not *C. difficile*)
	Atypical: None	**Atypical:** None	**Atypical:** None	**Atypical:** None
Spectrum of Activity Summary	Ertapenem does not cover *Pseudomonas, Acinetobacter* Imipenem/cilastatin has the best gram + coverage of the four (most reliable against *Enterococcus faecalis*) Meropenem/doripenem have the best gram – coverage Excellent anaerobic coverage with all carbapenems No atypical coverage in class			

(continued)

Antimicrobial	Ertapenem	Imipenem/Cilastatin	Meropenem	Doripenem
FDA-Approved Indications	• Complicated intra-abdominal infections, UTIs, SSTIs • CAP • Colorectal surgical prophylaxis • Acute pelvic infections	• Bacteremia • Gynecologic infections • Bone and joint infections • SSTIs • Complicated intra-abdominal infections • Infective endocarditis due to penicillinase-producing strains of *Staphylococcus aureus* • HCAP/VAP • Mixed infectious diseases (polymicrobial infections) • Complicated UTIs	• Bacterial meningitis • Complicated SSTIs • Complicated intra-abdominal infections	• Complicated intra-abdominal infections • Complicated UTIs • Pyelonephritis
Non-FDA-Approved Indications	Bacteremia associated with intravascular line	• Bacteremia associated with intravascular line • Cystic fibrosis (pulmonary exacerbations) • Febrile neutropenia • HCAP/VAP • Infective endocarditis due to penicillin-, aminoglycoside-, and vancomycin-resistant *Enterococcus faecalis*	• Bacteremia associated with an intravascular line • Cystic fibrosis (pulmonary exacerbations) • Febrile neutropenia • HCAP/VAP	• Bacteremia associated with an intravascular line
Pharmacodynamics	T>MIC; rapidly bactericidal, and prolonged PAE for gram + and − organisms			
Pharmacokinetics	Renal			
Distribution	Tissues—variable Body fluids—readily CSF—minimal (↑ with inflamed meninges) Placenta—crosses			

Adverse Effects	Generally well tolerated Cross-reactivity with penicillin allergy <1% *Clostridium difficile* infection			
	>5%: nausea, diarrhea, phlebitis, headache, ↑LFT 0.5%: seizures*	~3%: phlebitis ≤2%: diarrhea, nausea, and vomiting <1%: seizures*	≤8%: injection site inflammation, headache, constipation, diarrhea, nausea, vomiting, and seizures (<0.7%)	≥5%: phlebitis, diarrhea, nausea, rash, headache Seizure (unknown incidence)*, interstitial pneumonitis with inhaled doripenem
Drug Interactions	All carbapenems may ↑ valproic acid serum concentrations to below therapeutic levels resulting in breakthrough seizures. Concomitant use not recommended. If used, consider an alternative anticonvulsant and/or closely monitor valproic acid levels. Probenecid increases all carbapenem serum concentrations. Concomitant use should be avoided.			
		Ganciclovir and valganciclovir—concomitant use with imipenem/cilastatin may result in CNS toxicity (seizures)		
Dose Renal dose adjustments required. Refer to renal dosing table.	1 g IV Q24h	250–1,000 mg Q6–8h Dosing based on imipenem component	1 g IV Q8h (2 g for serious or CNS infections)	500 mg Q8h
Monitoring	Renal function Allergic reactions			
Resistance Mechanisms	Combination of reduced permeability due to porin loss and expression of AmpC-type enzymes or other ESBLs Efflux pumps Carbapenemases (carbapenem hydrolyzing β-lactamases)—plasmid mediated			

(continued)

Antimicrobial	Ertapenem	Imipenem/Cilastatin	Meropenem	Doripenem
Comments	* Mechanism of carbapenem-associated risk of seizures is due to interaction with the GABAa receptor. It depends primarily on the side chain on the second carbon atom in the carbapenem nucleus. The more basic the side chain, the better binding affinity which may result in increased seizure activity. The meropenem side chain is much less basic than imipenem/cilastatin. Risk with all carbapenems is also increased when dose is not adjusted accordingly for patients' renal function.			
	For obese patients (BMI ≥40), 1 g Q24h may be inadequate. Consider dose increase or alternative antimicrobial.	Role of cilastatin—prevents renal metabolism of imipenem by inhibition of dehydropeptidase (DHP) and also prevents imipenem-induced nephrotoxicity	Meropenem and doripenem are not metabolized by DHP and thus do not require cilastatin.	

III.2.3 CEPHALOSPORINS

Antimicrobial	First-Generation	Second-Generation	Third-Generation	Fourth-Generation	Fifth-Generation	Cephalosporin/β-Lactamase Inhibitor
Examples	Cefadroxil (PO) Cefazolin (IV) Cephalexin (PO)	Cefaclor (PO) Cefotetan (IV) Cefoxitin (IV) Cefprozil (PO) Cefuroxime axetil (PO) Cefuroxime sodium (IV)	Cefdinir (PO) Cefditoren (PO) Cefixime (PO) Cefotaxime (IV) Cefpodoxime proxetil (PO) Ceftazidime (IV) Ceftriaxone (IV, IM)	Cefepime (IV)	Ceftaroline (IV)	Ceftazidime/ avibactam (IV) Ceftolozane/tazobactam (IV)
Mechanism of Action	Inhibits cell wall synthesis					β-lactamase inhibitor binds to β-lactamase, prevents it from breaking down cephalosporin Inhibits cell wall synthesis
Spectrum of Activity	Gram +: *Staphylococcus* (except MRSA and MRSE), *Streptococcus*	Gram +: *Staphylococcus* (coverage not as good as first-generation) and *Streptococcus* (slightly better than first-generation)	Gram +: *Staphylococcus* (No MRSA or MRSE) and *Streptococcus*	Gram +: *Staphylococcus* (No MRSA or MRSE) and *Streptococcus*	Gram +: *Staphylococcus* (including MRSA, MRSE, VRSA) and *Streptococcus*	Gram +: *Streptococcus*

(continued)

Antimicrobial	First-Generation	Second-Generation	Third-Generation	Fourth-Generation	Fifth-Generation	Cephalosporin/ β-Lactamase Inhibitor
Spectrum of Activity (Cont'd)	**Gram −:** *E. coli, Klebsiella,* and *Proteus mirabilis*	**Gram −:** *E. coli, Klebsiella, Proteus, Neisseria, Moraxella, H. influenzae*	**Gram −:** *E. coli, Klebsiella, Proteus, Neisseria, Moraxella, Haemophilus, Salmonella, Shigella* (Note: Most *Enterobacteriaceae* are covered)	**Gram −:** *Enterobacteriaceae, Moraxella, Haemophilus, Neisseria* Better gram (−) coverage than the third-generation, including *Pseudomonas* and stable against some AmpC-producing β-lactamases	**Gram −:** Similar to third-generation; *Enterobacteriaceae, Haemophilus, Moraxella, Neisseria*	**Gram −:** *E. coli, Klebsiella, Proteus, Enterobacter, Citrobacter, Providencia, Pseudomonas*
	Anaerobes: *Actinomyces Lactobacillus, Peptococcus, Peptostreptococcus, P. acnes*	**Anaerobes:** *Peptococcus, Peptostreptococcus, P. acnes,* cefoxitin and cefotetan have broad anaerobic coverage including *B. fragilis*; however, resistance is increasing	**Anaerobes:** *Peptococcus, Peptostreptococcus, P. acnes,* cefotaxime and cefoperazone have some gram-negative anaerobic activity; however, not *B. fragilis*	**Anaerobes:** No reliable coverage	**Anaerobes:** No reliable coverage	**Anaerobes:** Broad including *B. fragilis* (ceftolozane/ tazobactam only)
	Atypical: None	**Atypical:** None	**Atypical:** None	**Atypical:** None	**Atypical:** None	**Atypical:** None
Spectrum of Activity Summary	Ceftaroline is the only cephalosporin with MRSA activity. No enterococcal activity. No antipseudomonal activity across the class. In general, as you increase in generation you gain better gram-negative activity. Ceftazidime, cefepime, ceftazidime/avibactam, and ceftolozane/tazobactam cover *Pseudomonas*. Cefoxitin, cefotetan, cefotaxime, and cefoperazone have good anaerobic activity. Ceftazidime/avibactam and ceftolozane/tazobactam have activity against some carbapenemase-producing organisms.					

FDA-Approved Indications	• Bacteremia • Cholangitis (susceptible organisms only) • Endocarditis • Osteomyelitis • SSTI • Surgical prophylaxis • URTI • UTI	• Intra-abdominal infections (+/−) • LRTI • Osteomyelitis • PID • SSTI • URTI • UTI	• Bacterial meningitis • Gonorrhea • Intra-abdominal infection • LRTI • Osteomyelitis • PID • SSTI • URTI • UTI	• Febrile neutropenia • Intra-abdominal infection • LRTI • SSTI • UTI	• CAP • SSTI	Complicated intra-abdominal infections Complicated UTI
Non-FDA-Approved Indications	• Other infections caused by Group A *Streptococcus* or MSSA	• *N. gonorrhoeae* (no longer recommended) • Surgical wound infections	• Bacteremia • Bacterial endocarditis • Diabetic foot infections • Febrile neutropenia (ceftazidime) • Intra-abdominal infection • Lyme disease • Salmonella infection	• Bacteremia • Bacterial endocarditis • Bacterial meningitis • Peritonitis (PD-associated)		
Pharmacodynamics	T>MIC; bactericidal, and + PAE (mostly for gram + organisms)					
Pharmacokinetics	Renal elimination	Renal elimination	Renal elimination except for ceftriaxone (renal and bile) and cefoperazone (biliary)	Renal elimination	Metabolized by phosphatase enzyme and hydrolysis and renally excreted	Renal elimination

(continued)

Antimicrobial	First-Generation	Second-Generation	Third-Generation	Fourth-Generation	Fifth-Generation	Cephalosporin/ β-Lactamase Inhibitor
Distribution	Body fluids—readily CSF—minimal (↑ with inflamed meninges) Tissues—readily	Body fluids—readily CSF—minimal (↑ with inflamed meninges) Tissues—readily	Body fluids—readily Bone—readily CSF—minimal (↑ with inflamed meninges) except readily with ceftriaxone, cefotaxime, and ceftazidime Tissues—readily	Body fluids—readily Bone—readily CSF—readily Tissues—readily	Body fluids— readily Tissues—readily	Body fluids—readily Tissues—readily
Adverse Effects	GI Rash	GI PO has MTT side chain—can cause ↑ PT and disulfiram reaction with EtOH Rash	Biliary sludging (pseudolithiasis)-ceftriaxone Bleeding, can impair vitamin K clotting factors (cefoperazone and ceftriaxone) Rash	GI HA Rash	Diarrhea Nausea Rash	GI HA Rash
	All cephalosporins: Usually well tolerated; allergic reaction (may be rash, hives, anaphylaxis), cross allergy with PCN is ~5% and less likely as generations increase; drug fever; seizures (very high doses in patients with renal insufficiency); positive Coombs' test without hemolysis; *Clostridium difficile* infection					
Drug Interactions	Low potential for drug interactions Probenecid Warfarin					

	Dose	Monitoring	Resistance Mechanisms	Comments
Cefazolin (IV) 1–2 g Q8h Cephalexin (PO) 250–500 mg Q6h Cefadroxil (PO) 500–1,000 mg Q12–24h			Altered penicillin-binding proteins Production of extended spectrum β-lactamases Efflux pumps Reduced permeability of bacterial membranes	Consider cefazolin 2–3 g doses for severe infections or patients >80 kg
Cefuroxime sodium (IV) 1 g Q8h Cefoxitin (IV) 2 g Q6h Cefotetan (IV) 1–2 g Q12h Cefuroxime axetil (PO) 500 mg Q12h Cefaclor (PO) 500 mg Q8h Cefprozil (PO) 500 mg Q12–24h	Concomitant use of ceftriaxone and IV calcium-containing solutions/products in neonates (≤ 28 day) is contraindicated Renal function			Cefoxitin and cefotetan have better activity against *Enterobacteriaceae* than the other second-generation cephalosporins
Ceftriaxone (IV) 1–2 g Q24h Cefotaxime (IV) 1–2 g Q12h Ceftazidime (IV) 1–2 g Q8h Cefixime (PO) 400 mg Q24h Cefdinir (PO) 300 mg Q12h or 600 mg Q24h Cefpodoxime proxetil (PO) 200–400 mg Q12h Cefditoren (PO) 400 mg Q12h				Avoid ceftriaxone in neonates; use cefotaxime as an alternative Consider ceftriaxone 2 g in severe infections or in patients >100 kg
Cefepime (IV) 0.5–2 g Q8–12h				Higher doses may be required for patients with severe infections or for those pathogens with elevated MICs
Ceftaroline (IV)—600 mg Q12h				
Ceftolozane/tazobactam (IV) 1.5 g Q8h (fifth-generation) Ceftazidime/avibactam (IV) 2.5 g Q8h				For both agents, must use in combination with metronidazole for treatment of intra-abdominal infections

III.2.4 FLUOROQUINOLONES

Antimicrobial	Older Generation Fluoroquinolones	Newer Generation Fluoroquinolones
Examples	Ciprofloxacin (IV, PO)— PO 250–750 mg Q12h; IV 200–400 mg Q12h Norfloxacin (PO)—400 mg Q12h Ofloxacin (PO, ophthalmic, otic)— PO 200–400 mg Q12h	Levofloxacin (IV, PO)— 250–750 mg Q24h Moxifloxacin (IV, PO, ophthalmic)— 400 mg Q24h
Mechanism of Action	Inhibits DNA gyrase and topoisomerase IV	
Spectrum of Activity	**Gram +:** *Staphylococcus* (increasing resistance), *Streptococcus* and *Enterococcus* are usually resistant	**Gram +:** *Staphylococcus* (usually MSSA and MSSE strains only), *Streptococcus* including *S. pneumoniae* *Enterococcus* is variable and not reliable
	Gram −: Broad including *Pseudomonas* (resistance increasing)	**Gram −:** Broad; levofloxacin has some coverage against *Pseudomonas aeruginosa*
	Anaerobes: None	**Anaerobes:** Moxifloxacin has broad coverage including *B. fragilis* (although resistance)
	Atypical: Yes (*Chlamydophilia pneumoniae, Mycoplasma pneumoniae, Legionella pneumoniae*)	**Atypical:** Yes (*Chlamydophila pneumoniae, Mycoplasma pneumoniae, Legionella pneumoniae*)
Spectrum of Activity Summary	Moxifloxacin and levofloxacin have pneumococcal coverage Moxifloxacin has anaerobic coverage Ciprofloxacin has the best pseudomonal coverage	
FDA-Approved Indications	Bone and joint infections Gonorrhea (increasing resistance rates) Infectious diarrhea Intra-abdominal infections LRTI Neutropenic fever, empiric therapy Post-exposure prophylaxis for inhalation anthrax Prostatitis Pyelonephritis SSTI Typhoid fever URTI UTI	
Non-FDA-Approved Indications	Cystic fibrosis exacerbations Endocarditis Meningitis Mycobacterium infections	

Antimicrobial	Older Generation Fluoroquinolones	Newer Generation Fluoroquinolones
Pharmacodynamics	AUC/MIC, bactericidal, +PAE	
Pharmacokinetics	Minimal hepatic metabolism, renal elimination Dosing adjustment required in renal dysfunction except moxifloxacin	
Distribution	Body fluids—variable Bone—readily CSF—good (↑ with inflamed meninges) Placenta—crosses Prostate—readily Tissues—readily	
Adverse Effects	C. difficile diarrhea Caution use in children—impaired bone/cartilage development CNS effects (HA, confusion, seizures) especially in elderly patients Elevated transaminases/hepatotoxicity (uncommon) GI upset Phototoxicity QT prolongation (ciprofloxacin least likely; moxifloxacin most likely) Rash or other severe allergic reactions Refractory hypoglycemia (moxifloxacin least likely, however, has also been implicated in hyperglycemia) Tendon rupture (most common Achilles, especially in patients >60 years, in transplant recipients, or concomitant corticosteroid use)	
Drug Interactions	Antiarrhythmic agents Chelation with multivalent cations; avoid co-administration or take FQ 2–4 h before or 4–8 h after Sevelamer Warfarin	
Monitoring	Renal function	
Resistance Mechanisms	Altered porin permeability (OmpF) Altered target site due to point mutations in topoisomerase IV and DNA gyrase Enzymatic degradation Increased drug efflux Plasmid-mediated gyrase inhibitor binding site protection (Qnr proteins)	
Comments	Ciprofloxacin not considered a "respiratory" fluoroquinolone due to lack of pneumococcal coverage Moxifloxacin does not have adequate urine concentrations and should not be used for UTIs Oral bioavailability for the majority of the quinolones/fluoroquinolones is > 90%; ciprofloxacin is less (~70–80%) The mechanism of hypoglycemia is the fluoroquinolones' ability to close K^+ ATP channels in the pancreatic β-cell resulting in the release of insulin	

III.2.5 FOSFOMYCIN

Antimicrobial	Fosfomycin
Mechanism of Action	Inhibits cell wall synthesis
Spectrum of Activity	**Gram +:** *Staphylococcus* spp. (including MRSA), *Streptococcus* spp., and *Enterococcus* spp. (including VRE)
	Gram −: *E. coli, Citrobacter* spp., *Proteus mirabilis, Klebsiella* spp. (including ESBL-producing isolates and CRE), *Pseudomonas* spp.
	Anaerobes: None
	Atypical: None
FDA-Approved Indications	Uncomplicated urinary tract infections
Non-FDA-Approved Indications	Complicated urinary tract infection without bacteremia
Pharmacodynamics	C_{max}/MIC, bactericidal, + PAE
Pharmacokinetics	Renal
Distribution	Bladder wall—readily Kidneys—readily Prostate—readily Seminal vesicles—readily
Adverse Effects	GI (diarrhea ~10%) HA
Drug Interactions	Antacids—reduces absorption of fosfomycin
Dose	3 g sachet PO × one dose If complicated, may repeat dose Q2–3 days (empty stomach preferred)
Monitoring	Resolution of symptoms; nothing specific to fosfomycin
Resistance Mechanisms	Chromosomal mutation minimizing fosfomycin transport into bacterial cell Plasmid-born inactivation
Comments	Mix in 120 mL of cool water until it dissolves; consume immediately Safe in pregnancy (Category B) Administer on an empty stomach

❖   ❖   ❖

III.2.6   GLYCOPEPTIDES/LIPOPEPTIDE

Antimicrobial	Glycopeptides	Lipopeptide
Examples	Vancomycin (IV, PO)	Daptomycin (IV)
Mechanism of Action	Disrupts bacterial cell membrane	Inhibits intracellular synthesis of DNA, RNA, and protein
Spectrum of Activity	**Gram +:** *Staphylococcus* spp. (including MRSA and MRSE), *Streptococcus* spp., *Enterococcus* spp.	**Gram +:** *Staphylococcus* spp. (including MRSA, MRSE, VISA, VRSA), *Streptococcus* spp., *Enterococcus* spp. (including VRE)
	Gram −: None	**Gram −:** None
	Anaerobes: Gram-positive anaerobic coverage	**Anaerobes:** Gram-positive anaerobic coverage
	Atypical: None	**Atypical:** None
FDA-Approved Indications	Bone and joint infections *Clostridium difficile* infection (oral formulation only) Infective endocarditis LRTIs	Bacteremia associated with intra-vascular line Complicated SSTIs *Staphylococcus aureus* bacteremia, including right-sided endocarditis
Non-FDA-Approved Indications	Febrile neutropenia Meningitis Peritoneal dialysis-associated peritonitis	Osteomyelitis Septic arthritis
Pharmacodynamics	AUC/MIC, bacteriostatic (may have cidal activity), + PAE	AUC/MIC or C_{max}/MIC, bactericidal for Staphylococcus and Streptococcus and bacterio-static for Enterococcus, + PAE
Pharmacokinetics	Renal	Renal
Distribution	CSF—variable Tissue—readily	Tissues—variable
Adverse Effects	Nephrotoxicity Ototoxicity Red Man Syndrome—infusion-related reaction (may be avoided by lengthening the infusion time) Thrombocytopenia	Arthralgia/myopathy CPK ↑ Eosinophlic pneumonia Injection site reaction Rash Rhabdomyolysis
Drug Interactions	Limited drug interactions Use caution when used concom-itantly with other nephrotoxic agents	Statins—increased potential for CPK ↑

Antimicrobial	Glycopeptides	Lipopeptide
Dose **Renal dose adjustments required. Refer to vancomycin pharmacokinetics and dosing**	Dosing frequency determined by renal function IV: 15–20 mg/kg Q8–48h PO: 125–500 mg PO Q6h	4 mg/kg/day for skin and soft tissue infections 6 mg/kg/day for bacteremia and endocarditis 8–10 mg/kg/day for severe infections
Monitoring	Renal function Serum trough concentrations: For *Staphylococcus aureus* with: • **MIC < 1 mcg/ml** goal trough = **10–15 mcg/mL** • **MIC = 1 mcg/mL** or severe infections (e.g., endocarditis, osteomyelitis, meningitis, hospital-acquired pneumonia, etc.) goal trough = **15–20 mcg/mL** • **MIC ≥ 2 mcg/mL**, utilize an alternative agent May consider baseline auditory testing depending on anticipated duration of therapy (>14 days) especially if used with concomitant ototoxic medications	CPK levels; weekly or more frequently in those patients on concomitant statin therapy, in patients with renal insufficiency, or in patients with CPK elevations Symptoms of muscle pain or weakness
Resistance Mechanisms	Alteration of peptidoglycan precursors (Van A, Van B, Van C phenotypes) Altered bacterial cell wall (thickening)	Increasing MIC Inoculum effect
Comments	Oral vancomycin for *Clostridium difficile* infection ONLY	Inactivated by surfactant; do not use to treat pneumonia Can be administered as an IV push or IVPB

III.2.7 GLYCYLCYCLINE

Antimicrobial	Glycylcycline
Example	Tigecycline (IV)
Mechanism of Action	Inhibits protein synthesis (30S subunit)
Spectrum of Activity	**Gram +:** *Staphylococcus* spp. (including CA-MRSA), *Streptococcus*, and *Enterococcus* (including VRE)
	Gram −: *Shigella, Serratia, Salmonella, Citrobacter, Enterobacter, E. coli, Klebsiella, H. influenzae, Stenotrophomonas, Acinetobacter,* including ESBL-producing organisms and CREs No pseudomonal coverage
	Anaerobes: Broad, including *B. fragilis*
	Atypical: Yes
FDA-Approved Indications	Community-acquired pneumonia (rarely used for CAP unless multiple drug allergies and/or contraindications to first-line agents) Complicated intra-abdominal infections Complicated SSTIs
Non-FDA-Approved Indications	Infections caused by multidrug-resistant organisms (including *Acinetobacter* and KPC-producing *Enterobacteraceae*)
Pharmacodynamics	AUC/MIC, bacteriostatic
Pharmacokinetics	Hepatic metabolism (adjust in severe hepatic disease); renal excretion (no renal dose adjustments)
Distribution	Tissues—extensive Body fluids—variable CSF—minimal/poor Placenta—crosses
Adverse Effects	Elevated LFTs GI (high incidence of nausea and vomiting; consider the addition of an antiemetic prior to dose to improve compliance) Hyperbilirubinemia Pancreatitis Tooth discoloration and inhibition of bone growth in children
Drug Interactions	Warfarin
Dose	100 mg load then 50 mg Q12h
Monitoring	Hepatic function
Resistance Mechanisms	Efflux pump Enzymatic resistance mechanism (TetX)
Comments	Highly protein bound (~80%) *Pseudomonas* is intrinsically resistant to tigecycline due to a multidrug efflux pump V_d 7–10 L/kg resulting in low serum concentrations (avoid for bacteremia)

III.2.8   KETOLIDE

Antimicrobial	Ketolide
Example	Telithromycin (PO)
Mechanism of Action	Inhibits protein synthesis by binding to domains II and V of 23S rRNA of the 50S ribosomal subunit
Spectrum of Activity	**Gram +:** *Staphylococcus aureus* (methicillin and erythromycin susceptible ONLY), *Streptococcus pneumoniae, Streptococcus pyogenes*
	Gram -: *H. influenzae, M. catarrhalis*
	Anaerobes: None
	Atypical: Yes
FDA-Approved Indications	Community-acquired pneumonia
Non-FDA-Approved Indications	Acute bacterial sinusitis and acute exacerbations of chronic bronchitis **Indications were removed from FDA-approval due to low benefit *versus* high risk of toxicity (specifically hepatotoxicity)**
Pharmacodynamics	AUC/MIC and C_{max}/MIC, bactericidal mostly, however, bacteriostatic against *S. aureus*, + PAE
Pharmacokinetics	70% hepatically metabolized; 13% renally eliminated
Distribution	Tissues– readily
Adverse Effects	Abnormal vision Acute hepatic failure GI Hepatitis QT prolongation
Drug Interactions	CYP3A4 and CYP1A2 substrate and CYP3A4 and CYP2D6 inhibitor, thus many drug interactions (e.g., midazolam, statins, rifampin, phenytoin, metoprolol, theophylline, digoxin, warfarin, etc.)
Dose	800 mg daily
Monitoring	Hepatic function Visual impairment symptoms
Resistance Mechanisms	Efflux pumps (Msr[A] and mef) Modification of the target site by methylation (*erm* gene)
Comments	**Black Box Warning:** Contraindicated in patients with myasthenia gravis due to reports of fatal and life-threatening respiratory failure

III.2.9   LINCOSAMIDE

Antimicrobial	Clindamycin
Mechanism of Action	Inhibits protein synthesis (50S subunit)
Spectrum of Activity	**Gram +:** *Staphylococcus* (including some CA-MRSA strains although increasing resistance) and *Streptococcus;* no Enterococcal coverage
	Gram −: None
	Anaerobes: Broad (NOT *C. difficile*); Increasing resistance in *B. fragilis*
	Atypical: None
FDA-Approved Indications	Acne vulgaris (topical) Bacterial vaginosis (vaginal) Pelvic infections Skin and soft tissue infections
Non-FDA-Approved Indications	MRSA skin and soft tissue infections or pneumonia (increasing resistance) Osteomyelitis *Pneumocystis jirovecii* pneumonia (+ primaquine) Sinusitis Toxoplasmosis (+ pyrimethamine and leucovorin)
Pharmacodynamics	AUC/MIC, bacteriostatic, + PAE
Pharmacokinetics	Metabolized in the liver (No dose adjustments made for renal function)
Distribution	Body fluids—readily Bone—readily CSF—none even with inflamed meninges Placenta—crosses Tissues—readily
Adverse Effects	Nausea, vomiting, and diarrhea *Clostridium difficile* infection Stevens-Johnson syndrome (rare)
Drug Interactions	Macrolides, streptogramins, oxazolidone, and chloramphenicol because they bind to the same ribosomal subunit, resulting in reduced activity Neuromuscular blocking agents
Dose	PO 300–450 mg Q6h; IV 600 mg Q6h or 900 mg Q8h
Monitoring	Diarrhea
Resistance Mechanisms	Efflux pumps Inactivating enzymes Modification of the ribosomal target (e.g., *erm*)
Comments	One of the most commonly implicated antimicrobials in *Clostridium difficile* infection Alternative for gram + infections when patient is PCN allergic Good (≥90%) oral bioavailability

III.2.10 LIPOGLYCOPEPTIDES

Antimicrobial	Dalbavancin	Oritavancin	Telavancin
Mechanism of Action	Inhibits cell wall synthesis	Inhibits cell wall synthesis Degrades integrity of cell membrane	Inhibits cell wall synthesis Degrades integrity of cell membrane
Spectrum of Activity	Gram +: Staphylococcus aureus (including MSSA and MRSA) and Streptococcus spp.	Gram +: Staphylococcus aureus (including MSSA and MRSA) and Streptococcus spp. and Enterococcus faecalis (only vancomycin-susceptible isolates)	Gram +: Staphylococcus aureus (including MSSA and MRSA) and Streptococcus spp. and Enterococcus faecalis (only vancomycin-susceptible isolates)
	Gram −: None	Gram −: None	Gram −: None
	Anaerobes: Gram-positive anaerobic coverage	Anaerobes: Gram-positive anaerobic coverage	Anaerobes: Gram-positive anaerobic coverage
	Atypical: None	Atypical: None	Atypical: None
FDA-Approved Indications	SSTIs	SSTIs	Complicated SSTIs HAP/VAP
Non-FDA-Approved Indications	Role in osteomyelitis, CAP, and catheter-related BSIs being evaluated	Role in pediatrics being evaluated	Role in pediatrics and BSI being evaluated
Pharmacodynamics	AUC/MIC, bactericidal, + PAE	AUC/MIC, bactericidal, + PAE	AUC/MIC, bactericidal, + PAE
Pharmacokinetics	Renal	Renal	Renal
Distribution	HIGHLY protein bound Tissues and fluids—excellent	HIGHLY protein bound Tissues and fluids—excellent	HIGHLY protein bound Placenta—crosses Tissues and fluids—excellent
Adverse Effects	GI HA Infusion-related reactions (Red Man Syndrome) LFT elevations	GI HA Infusion-related reactions (Red Man Syndrome) Falsely elevates aPTT for ~48 hours, PT and INR for 24 hours after administration	Altered taste (33%) Contraindicated in pregnancy Foamy urine (13%) GI (nausea 27%, vomiting 14%) Infusion-related reactions (Red Man Syndrome [lengthen infusion time to avoid])

	Dalbavancin	Oritavancin	Telavancin
Adverse Effects (*Cont'd*)			Insomnia Nephrotoxicity QT prolongation
Drug Interactions	None	Carbamazepine Phenytoin Unfractionated heparin up to 48 hours after administration Warfarin (not contraindicated; monitor)	Avoid concomitant QT-prolonging medications May increase INR, PT, aPTT, factor X assay, and activated clotting time
Dose	1,000 mg IV then 500 mg IV in 7 days CrCl <30 mL/min and NOT on HD: 750 mg followed by 375 mg	Single 1,200-mg dose over 3 hours IV infusion	10 mg/kg/day CrCl <50 mL/min: 7.5 mg/kg Q24h CrCl 10–30 mL/min: 10 mg/kg Q48h
Monitoring	Renal and hepatic function	Renal function Signs/symptoms of bleeding Signs/symptoms of osteomyelitis	Renal function QT interval Pregnancy test prior to use in women of child-bearing potential
Resistance Mechanisms	Alteration of peptidoglycan precursors (Van A phenotypes)	Alteration of peptidoglycan precursors (Van A phenotypes)	Alteration of peptidoglycan precursors (Van A phenotypes)
Comments	Reconstitute 500-mL vial using 25 mL of sterile water for injection. Alternate gentle swirling and inversion to prevent foaming. ONLY 5% Dextrose is an appropriate final diluent. Do **NOT** use 0.9% Normal Saline as this will result in precipitation of dalbavancin Final concentration 1 mg/mL and 5 mg/mL	Three 400-mg vials are used to prepare a single 1,200-mg dose Add 40 mL of sterile water for injection to each vial and gently swirl to prevent foaming during reconstitution. ONLY 5% Dextrose is an appropriate final diluent. Do **NOT** use 0.9% Normal Saline as this will result in precipitation of oritavancin Withdraw 120 mL from D5W 1,000 mL for infusion, and then add contents of three 40-mL vials of reconstituted oritavancin in sterile water	**Black box warning:** women of childbearing potential should have a serum pregnancy test prior to administration. Based on animal data, telavancin may cause fetal harm; avoid in pregnancy **Black box warning:** for renal insufficiency. Formulation of telavancin contains the solubilizer cyclodextrin, which may accumulate in patients with renal dysfunction Hazardous medication precautions

III.2.11 MACROLIDES

Antimicrobial	First-Generation Macrolide	Second-Generation Macrolide
Example	Erythromycin (IV, PO) IV 0.5–1 g Q6h PO 250–500 mg Q6h	Azithromycin (IV, PO)—250–500 mg Q24h Clarithromycin (PO)—250–500 mg Q12h
Mechanism of Action	Inhibits protein synthesis (50s subunit)	
Spectrum of Activity	**Gram +:** *Staphylococcus* (MSSA, MSSE only, however, considerable resistance) and *Streptococcus* (especially *S. pneumoniae* and *S. pyogenes*)	**Gram +:** *Staphylococcus* (MSSA, MSSE only, however, considerable resistance) and *Streptococcus* (especially *S. pneumoniae* and *S. pyogenes*) however, considerable *S. pneumoniae* resistance
	Gram −: Limited (*Moraxella, Bordetella pertussis, H. pylori, N. meningitides, N. gonorrhea* [increasing resistance])	**Gram −:** *N. meningitidis, H. influenzae* (+/−), *N. gonorrhea, Bordetella pertussis, Moraxella, Pasturella multocida, Bartonella, Campylobacter*
	Anaerobes: Minimal (mostly gram-positive anaerobes)	**Anaerobes:** Minimal (mostly gram-positive anaerobes)
	Atypical: Yes (should not be used for *Legionella*)	**Atypical:** Yes
	Other: +/− *M. avium*	**Other:** Atypical mycobacteria, *Chlamydia trachomatis* (azithromycin)
FDA-Approved Indications	Acne vulgaris Amebiasis (*Entamoeba histolytica*) Listeriosis LRTI (community-acquired) Newborn conjunctivitis (*Chlamydia trachomatis*) Pertussis PID Rheumatic fever prophylaxis (PCN allergy) SSTI (mild) Surgical bowel preparation Syphilis (alternative to PCN in PCN allergy; azithromycin preferred) Urethritis (uncomplicated) URTI	*H. pylori* infections as part of combination therapy (clarithromycin only) LRTI (community-acquired) *Mycobacterium avium* infections and prophylaxis SSTI (mild) URTI

Antimicrobial	First-Generation Macrolide	Second-Generation Macrolide
Non-FDA-Approved Indications	Gastroparesis Lyme disease	Bartonella Lyme disease Pertussis
Pharmacodynamics	AUC/MIC, bacteriostatic, +PAE	
Pharmacokinetics	Hepatic metabolism	
Distribution	Body fluids—readily CSF—poor Placenta—crosses Tissues—readily	
Adverse Effects	GI upset (especially erythromycin) Hepatitis Metallic taste (especially clarithromycin) Phlebitis (especially IV erythromycin) QT prolongation/torsades de pointes (may lead to sudden death; erythromycin most likely); patients at highest risk for QT-prolongation include those with known risk factors such as preexisting QT prolongation, hypokalemia, or hypomagnesemia, bradycardia, or concomitant antiarrhythmics Reversible ototoxicity (especially IV erythromycin)	
Drug Interactions	Inhibits CYP1A2 and 3A4; thus many possible drug interactions (e.g., calcium channel blockers; antiarrhythmics; carbamazepine; phenytoin; theophylline; warfarin; statins, azoles) Substrate of CYP2B6	Substrate and inhibitor of CYP3A4; thus many possible drug interactions More interaction potential with clarithromycin versus azithromycin
Monitoring	Hepatic function	
Resistance Mechanisms	Modification of the target site by methylation (*erm* gene) Efflux pumps (Msr[A] and mef) Antimicrobial inactivation by phosphorylases or esterases	
Comments	Azithromycin has a very long $t_{1/2}$ Erythromycin best on empty stomach Erythromycin should not be used for MAC treatment/prophylaxis Excellent oral bioavailability Macrolides also hyperproduce algination, exist as a biofilm, and inhibit pseudomonal biofilm formation (important for chronic respiratory conditions such as cystic fibrosis and bronchiectasis) Macrolides have been shown to demonstrate immunomodulatory effects Erthromycin use is commonly reserved as a gastric motility agent (diabetes-associated gastroparesis)	

III.2.12 MONOBACTAMS

Antimicrobial	Aztreonam (IV, INH)
Mechanism of Action	Inhibits cell wall synthesis
Spectrum of Activity	**Gram +:** None
	Gram −: Broad spectrum including *Pseudomonas* (although increasing rates of pseudomonal resistance) and lacks coverage of ESBL-producing organisms
	Anaerobes: None
	Atypical: None
FDA-Approved Indications	Cystic fibrosis exacerbations Gram-negative infections: pneumonia; skin and soft tissue; urinary tract, gynecologic, and intra-abdominal infections
Non-FDA-Approved Indications	Diabetic foot infections Osteomyelitis
Pharmacodynamics	T>MIC; bactericidal, and + PAE
Pharmacokinetics	Renal
Distribution	Body fluids—readily CSF—minimal (↑ with inflamed meninges) Placenta—crosses Tissues—readily
Adverse Effects	Minimal—**NO cross allergy with PCN**
Drug Interactions	Probenecid—↑ aztreonam
Dose	1–2 g Q8h IVPB Consider using 2 g for obese patients and severe infections 75 mg INH b/w 75 mg and TID (at least four hours apart)
Monitoring	Renal function
Resistance Mechanisms	Efflux pumps Production of extended spectrum β-lactamases Reduced permeability due to porin loss
Comments	Inhaled aztreonam can be used for CF patients; however, the lysine salt formulation should be utilized as the IV formulation contains arginine, which causes airway inflammation. Typically reserved for those patients with a documented PCN allergy Increasing resistance, especially *Pseudomonas*

III.2.13 NITROFURANS

Antimicrobial	Nitrofurans
Examples	Macrodantin Nitrofurantoin macrocrystals
Mechanism of Action	Inhibits bacterial enzymes Attacks bacterial ribosomal proteins resulting in complete inhibition of bacterial protein synthesis
Spectrum of Activity	**Gram +:** *Staphylococcus* spp., *Streptococcus* spp., and *Enterococcus* spp.
	Gram −: *E. coli*, +/− *Enterobacter*, +/− *Citrobacter*, +/− *Klebsiella* (including some ESBL-producing isolates)
	Anaerobes: None
	Atypical: None
FDA-Approved Indications	Uncomplicated UTIs
Non-FDA-Approved Indications	Recurrent UTIs UTIs in pregnancy UTI prophylaxis
Pharmacodynamics	Unknown
Pharmacokinetics	Hepatic metabolism with renal excretion
Distribution	Serum—poor Tissues—poor Urine and kidneys—extensive
Adverse Effects	GI (macrocrystal formulation better tolerated) Hemolytic anemia (especially with G6PD deficiency) Hepatitis (can mimic autoimmune hepatitis) Hypersensitivity with pulmonary symptoms (fever, cough, dyspnea potentially with infiltrate and eosinophilia) Pancreatitis Peripheral neuropathy (long-term use) Pulmonary fibrosis (long-term use) Rash
Drug Interactions	Norfloxacin (antagonism) Other concomitant drugs causing neurotoxicity
Dose	50–100 mg Q6h or monohydrate/macrocrystals 100 mg Q12h
Monitoring	Pulmonary function tests and chest radiograph if long-term therapy Renal and hepatic function
Resistance Mechanisms	Chromosomal and plasmid-born genes
Comments	Avoid in patients with CrCl 40–60 mL/min as drug will concentrate in the serum due to lack of renal excretion resulting in inadequate drug concentrations at the infection site and increased risk of toxicity Duration of therapy for uncomplicated UTI with nitrofurantoin should be 5 days Does not induce as much resistance as and retains susceptibility compared to other commonly used agents for UTIs such as fluoroquinolones and β-lactams.

III.2.14   NITROIMIDAZOLE

Antimicrobial	Nitroimidazole
Example	Metronidazole (IV, PO, vaginal, topical)
Mechanism of Action	Interferes with DNA activity
Spectrum of Activity	**Gram +:** None
	Gram −: None
	Anaerobes: Broad, including *B. fragilis, Clostridium difficile*
	Atypical: None
FDA-Approved Indications	Acne rosacea Anaerobic infections—abscesses, meningitis, intra-abdominal infections, skin and soft tissue infections, bone and joint infections, endocarditis, gynecologic infections, lower respiratory tract infections, etc. Bacterial vaginosis *H. pylori* (as part of combination therapy) Trichomoniasis
Non-FDA-Approved Indications	*Clostridium difficile* infection Giardiasis Periodontal disease Surgical prophylaxis
Pharmacodynamics	C_{max}/MIC and AUC/MIC, rapidly bactericidal, +PAE
Pharmacokinetics	Metabolized in liver, eliminated renally
Distribution	CSF—well ($\uparrow$ with inflamed meninges) Placenta—crosses Tissues, body fluids, and bone—readily
Adverse Effects	Disulfiram reaction (avoid ethanol) GI Headache Metallic taste Peripheral neuropathy (with prolonged use; mechanism unknown, however, may involve metronidazole binding to neuronal RNA in nerve cells which may inhibit neuronal protein synthesis and result in peripheral axonal degeneration) Seizures (rare)
Drug Interactions	Amiodarone Barbiturates Busulfan Disulfiram Fluorouracil Lithium Mycophenolate Phenytoin Ritonavir/lopinavir liquid Tipranavir Warfarin

Antimicrobial	Nitroimidazole
Dose	500 mg Q6–8h (usually Q8h) ER formulation 750 mg Q12h 2 g once for trichomoniasis
Monitoring	Signs and symptoms of neuropathy
Resistance Mechanisms	Excellent oral bioavailability Reduction of pyruvate: ferredoxin oxidoreductase (PFOR) and hydrogenase, which limits cellular uptake and results in subsequent inactivation Resistance is rare

III.2.15 OXAZOLIDINONES

Antimicrobial	Oxazolidinones	
Example	Linezolid (IV, PO)	Tedizolid (IV, PO)
Mechanism of Action	Inhibits protein synthesis (50S subunit)	
Spectrum of Activity	**Gram +:** Broad including MRSA, MRSE, VRE	**Gram +:** *Staphylococcus* spp. including MRSA, *Streptococcus* spp., *Enterococcus* spp.
	Gram –: None	**Gram –:** None
	Anaerobes: Yes (including some gram negative anaerobes)	**Anaerobes:**
	Atypical: Yes	**Atypical:** Yes
FDA-Approved Indications	Community-acquired pneumonia Complicated and uncomplicated SSTIs Hospital-acquired pneumonia Vancomycin-resistant *Enterococcus faecium* infections	Acute bacterial SSTIs
Non-FDA-Approved Indications	Bacteremia associated with intravascular line (generally not recommended) Joint infections Osteomyelitis	—
Pharmacodynamics	AUC/MIC and t>MIC, bacteriostatic, short PAE	AUC/MIC, bacteriostatic, short PAE
Pharmacokinetics	Minimal hepatic metabolism; 30% unchanged and 10-40% as metabolites renally eliminated	Tedizolid phosphate is a prodrug that is converted by phosphatases to tedizolid, the microbiologically active moiety; eliminated via liver 82% feces and 18% urine

Antimicrobial	Oxazolidinones	
Distribution	Bone—good CSF—good Tissues—readily	Tissues—readily
Adverse Effects	Bone marrow suppression [thrombo-cytopenia/anemia]; especially with >14 days of therapy) Gl Lactic acidosis (rare) Malaise Neuropathy (peripheral/optic)—with prolonged use Serotonin syndrome (especially with concomitant serotonergic agents)	Caution in neutropenic patients (decreased efficacy) Gl Headache Only studied in clinical trials for a duration of 6 days; watch for same adverse effects as linezolid if used for longer duration
Drug interactions	Linezolid is a reversible, nonselective monoamine oxidase inhibitor Buspirone Meperidine Serotonin 5-HT1 receptor agonists SSRIs Tricyclic antidepressants	Tedizolid is a reversible inhibitor of monoamine oxidase; in clinical trials, patients receiving concomitant SSRIs, tricyclic antidepressants, serotonin 5-HT1 receptor agonists, meperidine, or buspirone were excluded thus the safety of co-administration is unknown
Dose	600 mg Q12h	200 mg Q24h
Monitoring	CBC with differential weekly Myelosuppression Persistent diarrhea and/or nausea/vomiting (progressing to lactic acidosis) Seizure activity Serotonin syndrome (especially with concomitant serotonergic agents) Signs and symptoms of peripheral neuropathy Visual impairment (especially with long-term use)	CBC with differential
Resistance Mechanisms	Resistance is oftentimes associated with prolonged use of linezolid Target site mutation (e.g., *cfr* gene)	Potentially target site mutation (e.g., *cfr* gene) with other chromosomal mutations
Comments	100% bioavailability CBC with differential weekly especially if long-term use is expected Consider q8h dosing for severe infections in morbidly obese patients	Excellent bioavailability

III.2.16 PENICILLINS

Antimicrobial	Penicillin	Anti-Staphylococcal (Penicillinase-Resistant)	Aminopenicillin	Anti-Pseudomonal	β-Lactam/β-Lactamase Inhibitor
Examples	Penicillin G (IV or PO)— IV 1–4 million units Q4h Penicillin VK PO— 250–500 mg Q6h	Nafcillin (IV) Oxacillin (IV) Dicloxacillin (PO) IV 1–2 g Q4–6h PO 250–500 mg Q6h	Ampicillin (IV, PO)— IV 1–2 g Q4–6h PO 250–500 mg Q6h Amoxicillin PO 250–500 mg Q8h	Carboxypenicillins: Ticarcillin (discontinued) Ureidopenicillins: Piperacillin IV 3–4 g Q6h	Ticarcillin/clavulanic acid IV 3.1 g Q4–6h Piperacillin/tazobactam IV 2.25–4.5 g Q6h Ampicillin/sulbactam IV 1.5–3 g Q6–8h Amoxicillin/clavulanic acid PO 250–500 mg Q8h or 875 mg Q12h
Mechanism of Action	Inhibits cell wall synthesis				β-lactamase inhibitor binds to β-lactamase, prevents it from breaking down penicillin Inhibits cell wall synthesis
Spectrum of Activity	Gram +: *Streptococcus, Enterococcus faecalis, +/– faecium* Gram–: *Neisseria meningitides* (penicillin G only), *Treponema pallidum, Pasturella*	Gram +: *Staphylococcus* spp. (no MRSA coverage) and *Streptococcus* spp. Does NOT cover *Enterococcus* Gram –: None	Gram +: *Streptococcus* spp. *Enterococcus, Listeria* Gram –: *E. coli* (at many institutions, up to 50% of isolates are resistant), *Proteus mirabilis*	Gram +: *Staphylococcus, Streptococcus, +/– Enterococcus* NOT as good as other penicillins against these Gram +s Gram –: Broad— including *Pseudomonas*	Gram +: *Staphylococcus, Streptococcus, Enterococcus* Ampicillin/sulbactam and amoxicillin/clavulanic acid have slightly better Enterococcal and anaerobic activity Gram –: Broad—including *Pseudomonas* Only ticarcillin/clavulanic acid and piperacillin/tazobactam have antipseudomonal activity

(continued)

Antimicrobial	Penicillin	Anti-Staphylococcal (Penicillinase-Resistant)	Aminopenicillin	Anti-Pseudomonal	β-Lactam/β-Lactamase Inhibitor
Spectrum of Activity (Cont'd)	**Anaerobes:** *Peptostreptococcus, Actinomyces, Clostridium non-difficile* **Atypical:** None	**Anaerobes:** *Peptostreptococcus* **Atypical:** None	*H. pylori* (amoxicillin), *Salmonella, Shigella* **Anaerobes:** Gram + anaerobes such as *Peptococcus, Peptostreptococcus, Clostridium non-difficile, Actinomyces* **Atypical:** None	**Anaerobes:** Broad—including *Bacteroides fragilis* and *Clostridium* spp. **Atypical:** None	*E. coli* is becoming increasingly resistant to ampicillin/sulbactam High-dose ampicillin/sulbactam has a role in the treatment of MDR *Acinetobacter baumannii* **Anaerobes:** Broad—including *Bacteroides fragilis* and *Clostridium* spp. **Atypical:** None
FDA-Approved Indications	• Actinomycosis • Anthrax (avoid as first-line) • Empyema • Endocarditis • Fusospirochetosis • Otitis media • *Pasteurella* infections • Pneumonia • Prophylaxis for: glomerulonephritis, rheumatic fever, rheumatic heart disease, rheumatic	• Endocarditis (susceptible staphylococcal strains) • Staphylococcal infections	• Diverticulitis • Endocarditis • Enteric infections • *H. pylori* (amoxicillin—part of combination therapy) • Meningitis • Otitis media • Respiratory tract infections • Streptococcal infections • UTI	• Bacteremia • Gonorrhea • Gynecological infections • Intra-abdominal infections • Intra-articular infections • Osteomyelitis • Pneumonia • Skin and soft tissue infections • UTI	• Gynecologic infections (pelvic inflammatory disease) • Pneumonia • Intra-abdominal infections (peritonitis, appendicitis)

Non-FDA-Approved Indications	• Rat bite fever • SSTI • Syphilis (benzathine PCN) • URTI	• Gas gangrene • Leptosporosis • Lyme disease • Necrotizing faciitis • *Neisseria meningitidis* • Neurosyphilis (benzathine PCN)	• Staphylococcal (MSSA) infections such as: osteomyelitis, skin and soft tissue infections, bacteremia, catheter-related infections, septic arthritis	• Community-acquired meningitis (*Listeria* coverage) • Enteric infections (*Vibrio cholera*) • Enterococcal endocarditis • *Enterococcus* coverage • Intra-abdominal abscess (part of combination therapy) • Lyme disease • Pharyngitis	• Febrile neutropenia	• Febrile neutropenia • Bacteremia
Pharmaco-dynamics	$T > MIC$; rapidly bactericidal, and minimal PAE for gram + organisms only					
Pharmaco-kinetics	Renal	Biliary Dose adjust if both severe renal AND hepatic dysfunction	Renal (amoxicillin has better GI absorption)	Renal		Renal

(continued)

Antimicrobial	Penicillin	Anti-Staphylococcal (Penicillinase-Resistant)	Aminopenicillin	Anti-Pseudomonal	β-Lactam/β-Lactamase Inhibitor
Distribution	Body fluids—readily Bone CSF—minimal (↑ with inflamed meninges) Placenta—crosses Tissues—variable	Body fluids—readily Bone—variable CSF—minimal (↑ with inflamed meninges) Placenta—crosses Tissues—variable	Body fluids—readily Bone—readily CSF—minimal (↑ with inflamed meninges) Placenta—crosses Tissues—variable	Body fluids—readily CSF—minimal (↑ with inflamed meninges) Placenta—crosses Tissues—variable	Body fluids—readily CSF—minimal (↑ with inflamed meninges) Placenta—crosses Tissues—variable
Adverse Effects	Allergic reaction (may be rash, hives, anaphylaxis) / Clostridium difficile infection / Drug fever / Jarisch-Herxheimer reaction / Seizures (very high doses in patients with renal insufficiency)				
	Interstitial nephritis (rare)	Nausea, vomiting, diarrhea, LFT elevation (especially oxacillin), rash (more likely with oxacillin), phlebitis, interstitial nephritis	Diarrhea (less with amoxicillin), rash	Generally well tolerated GI intolerance	GI (diarrhea, nausea, cramping), especially amoxicillin/ clavulanate
Drug Interactions	Probenecid—increased PCN concentrations; may be beneficial if high concentrations needed				
	Methotrexate Tetracyclines— antagonism	Decreased effect of warfarin	Allopurinol Methotrexate	Allopurinol Methotrexate Tetracyclines	
Monitoring	Allergic reaction Hepatic function (oxacillin) Renal function				

Resistance Mechanisms	Altered penicillin binding proteins Efflux pumps Production of extended spectrum β-lactamases Reduced permeability of bacterial membranes		
Comments	Benzathine PCN (Bicillin LA) and benzathine procaine (Bicillin CR) PCN are **NOT** interchangeable 250 mg = 400 K units 1.7 mEq Na or K per million unit	↑ Incidence of rash with ampicillin if patient has virus or is taking allopurinol Amoxicillin has considerably better oral absorption than ampicillin Ampicillin has short stability Production of β-lactamases by gram-negative organisms are barriers to use	
	Oxacillin is more likely to cause hepatotoxicity; reversible with discontinuation Nafcillin more likely than oxacillin to cause interstitial nephritis With high dose for an extended duration, potassium wasting may occur with nafcillin and oxacillin Dicloxacillin has best F (~75%) Oxacillin contains 2.5 mEq of sodium per gram and nafcillin contains 2.9 mEq of sodium per gram. Consider this sodium load, especially in patients with conditions requiring sodium restriction such as heart failure	Piperacillin 1 g = 1.85 mEq Na	Watch Na overload; piperacillin/tazobactam 1 g = 2.79 mEq Na

III.2.17 POLYMYXINS

Antimicrobial	Polymyxins (IV, otic, ophthalmic, INH)	
Examples	Polymyxin E (colistin, colistimethate sodium)	Polymyxin B
Mechanism of Action	Disrupts bacterial cell membrane	
Spectrum of Activity	**Gram +:** None	
	Gram −: *P. aeruginosa, K. pneumoniae, H. influenzae, E. coli, Entero-bacter* spp., *Acinetobacter* spp.	
	Anaerobes: None	
	Atypical: None	
FDA-Approved Indications	Gram-negative infections (usually MDROs) Meningitis Ocular infections	
Non-FDA-Approved Indications	Respiratory tract infections Sepsis	Superficial topical infections Surgical irrigation Irrigation of bladder
Pharmacodynamics	AUC/MIC, bactericidal, + PAE	
Pharmacokinetics	Renal elimination	
Distribution	Tissues—readily CSF—variable	
Adverse Effects	Nephrotoxicity (requires renal dose adjustment); dose dependent and usually reversible Neurotoxicity (paresthesia, dizziness, vertigo, blurred vision, slurred speech, ataxia) Neurotoxicity and nephrotoxicity much less than originally reported with historic data Phlebitis INH can cause possible bronchospasm and ARDS (especially when not used immediately after preparation due to prodrug conversion to colistin)	
Drug Interactions	Neuromuscular blockers—avoid co-administration when possible; if needed, monitor neuromuscular function closely	
Dose	Polymyxin E IV 2.5–5 mg/kg given in 2–3 divided doses (consider a loading dose of 5–7.5 mg/kg in critically ill patients in the ICU) Intraventricular: 5–10 mg Q12h INH: 75 mg in 3 mL NS via nebulizer Q12h; prepare immediately prior to use Otic: 1–2 drops Q6–8h to affected ear	Polymyxin B 15,000–25,000 units/kg/day given in 2 divided doses (maximum daily dose of 2,000,000 units) Bladder irrigation: continuous or rinse in the urinary bladder for up to 10 days using 20 mg (equal to 200,000 units) added to 1 L of normal saline; usually no more than 1 L is used per day unless urine flow rate is high; administration rate is adjusted to patient's urine output

Antimicrobial	Polymyxins (IV, otic, ophthalmic, INH)	
Dose		Intraventricular: 50,000 units once daily for 3–4 days then, every other day Ophthalmic: 1–3 drops Q3h (maximum of 6 doses/day) to affected eye Otic: 1–2 drops 3–4 times daily Topical irrigation: 500,000 units/L normal saline

Monitoring	Systemic use:
	  Renal function
	  CNS toxicity	

Resistance Mechanisms	Heteroresistance reported Uncommon; however, resistance increasing	
Comments	Prodrug: colistimethate sodium is hydrolyzed to active colistin Unit conversion: colistin sulfate 1 mg = 30,000 units; colistin methanesulfonate 2.5 mg = 30,000 units) Inactive against some Gram– (*Proteus* spp., *Burkholderia* spp., *Providencia* spp., *Serratia* spp., and Gram (–) cocci) Usually reserved for multidrug-resistant organisms For organisms with an MIC ≥ 2 mcg/mL, unlikely to obtain clinically effective concentrations	Dose conversion: 1 mg = 10,000 units IM administration not recommended due to pain at injection site Inactive against some Gram– (*Proteus* spp., *Burkholderia* spp., *Providencia* spp., *Serratia* spp., and Gram– cocci) Usually reserved for multidrug-resistant organisms For organisms with an MIC ≥ 2 mcg/mL, unlikely to obtain clinically effective concentrations

III.2.18   STREPTOGRAMIN

Antimicrobial	Streptogramin
Example	Quinupristin/dalfopristin (IV)
Mechanism of Action	Inhibits protein synthesis (50S subunit)
Spectrum of Activity	**Gram +:** *Staphylococcus* (MSSA, MRSA, MSSE, MRSE), *Streptococcus* spp., *Enterococcus faecium* (including VRE)
	Gram −: *Moraxella, H. influenzae*
	Anaerobes: None
	Atypical: Yes
FDA-Approved Indications	Complicated skin and soft tissue infections
Non-FDA-Approved Indications	Infective endocarditis (not recommended due to inadequate clearance of bacteremia) MRSA infections Vancomycin-resistant *Enterococcus faecium* infections
Pharmacodynamics	AUC/MIC, bactericidal against *Staphylococcus* and *Streptococcus* (due to synergism between the two agents), bacteriostatic against *E. faecium*, + PAE
Pharmacokinetics	Metabolism in liver by non-enzymatic reactions Feces, urine
Distribution	Tissues—readily
Adverse Effects	Arthritis/myalgia Conjugated hyperbilirubinemia and hyperbilirubinemia (asymptomatic) GI Phlebitis/injection site reactions Thrombophlebitis
Drug Interactions	Quinupristin—weak CYP3A4 inhibitor CYP3A4 substrates
Dose	7.5 mg/kg Q8h (Q12h for skin and soft tissue infections)
Monitoring	Bilirubin levels
Resistance Mechanisms	Drug inactivation by enzymes Efflux or active transport Plasmid-coded conformational alterations in ribosomal target binding site
Comments	*Enterococcus faecalis* is intrinsically resistant to dalfopristin due to an efflux pump; thus, most *E. faecalis* are resistant Infuse by central venous catheter Myalgia may preclude use Rarely used due to adverse effects (typically salvage)

III.2.19   SULFONAMIDE

Antimicrobial	Sulfonamide
Example	Sulfamethoxazole/trimethoprim (TMP/SMX) (IV, PO)
Mechanism of Action	SMX inhibits dihydrofolic acid formation from PABA TMP inhibits dihydrofolic acid reduction to tetrahydrofolate
Spectrum of Activity	**Gram +:** *Staphylococcus* spp. (including CA-MRSA), *Streptococcus* (resistance increasing), *Nocardia* spp.
	Gram −: *Enterobacteriaceae* (except *Providencia* are resistant and *E. coli* resistance increasing), *H. influenzae, Stenotrophomonas*
	Anaerobes: Unreliable
	Atypical: None
	Other: Protozoa such as *Pneumocystis jeroveci* (PJP) and *Toxoplasma gondii*
FDA-Approved Indications	AECB Otitis media *Pneumocystis jirovecii* pneumonia infection/prophylaxis Traveler's diarrhea (*Shigellosis*) UTIs
Non-FDA-Approved Indications	*Isospora, Cyclospora* infections *Listeria* infections (PCN allergy) Meningitis *Nocardia* infections SSTIs (CA-MRSA) *Stenotrophomonas* infections *Toxoplasma gondii* infections/prophylaxis UTI prophylaxis
Pharmacodynamics	T>MIC, bacteriostatic (bactericidal against *Listeria*)
Pharmacokinetics	Metabolized in liver via N-acetylation and glucuronidation, eliminated renally
Distribution	Body fluids—readily CSF—good Tissues—readily
Adverse Effects	Bone marrow suppression GI (especially with higher doses) Hepatitis Hyperkalemia (reversible) Kernicterus in newborns LFT elevations Nephrotoxicity Pancreatitis Photosensitivity Rash and pruritis (although less common, may include Stevens-Johnson syndrome, TEN, and erythema multiforme)

Antimicrobial	Sulfonamide
Drug Interactions	Dofetilide Methotrexate Pimozide Terfenadine Thioridazine Warfarin
Dose	10–20 mg/kg/day (dose based on trimethoprim component and actual body weight) in divided doses Higher doses are required for PJP treatment and CA-MRSA skin and soft tissue infections
Monitoring	CBC with differential Potassium Renal function
Resistance Mechanisms	Alterations in bacterial cell wall permeability Chromosomal mutations in the target genes that encode dihydropteroate synthetase and dihydrofolate reductase Modifications of the pathway for DNA synthesis Mutational loss of the ability of some bacteria to methylate deoxyuridylic acid to thymidylic acid bacteria dependent on external supply of thymidine Plasmid-mediated or transposon-mediated resistance (e.g., *sul* I, *sul* II)
Comments	Trimethoprim is structurally related to the potassium-sparing diuretics (triamterene and amiloride), thereby inhibiting sodium channels in the distal tubule resulting in hyperkalemia Excellent oral bioavailability Adverse effects are more common with higher treatment doses versus prophylactic doses

III.2.20 TETRACYCLINES

Antimicrobial	Tetracyclines
Examples	Doxycycline (IV, PO)—PO 50–100 mg Q12h; IV 100–200 mg Q12h Minocycline (IV, PO)—50–100 mg Q12h Tetracycline (PO)—PO 250–500 mg Q6h
Mechanism of Action	Inhibits protein synthesis (30S subunit) and blocking binding of aminoacyl transfer-RNA

Antimicrobial	Tetracyclines
Spectrum of Activity	**Gram +:** *Staphylococcus* (including CA-MRSA), *Streptococcus* spp. (considerable resistance observed), *E. faecalis* (not first line), *Listeria* spp.
	Gram −: *Enterobacteriaceae* (not always reliable), *Vibrio* spp., *Yersinia pestis* (doxycycline), *Acinetobacter, Burkholderia cepacia* (minocycline), *Bartonella, Stenotrophomonas, Campylobacter* spp., *Chlamydia* spp., *Neisseria gonorrhoeae, H. pylori* (tetracycline)
	Anaerobes: Yes (not first line)
	Atypical: Yes
	Other: Spirochetes (Lyme disease and Borreliosis) and non-tubercular *Mycobacteria* spp., Rickettsiae (doxycycline), *Coxiella, Bacillus anthracis,* parasites (minocycline) (e.g., *Toxoplasma gondii, Trichomonas vaginalis, Entamoeba histolytica,* and *Giardia lamblia,* etc.)
FDA-Approved Indications	Acne vulgaris Actinomycoses Anthrax Bartonellosis Brucellosis Chancroid Chlamydial infection Cholera Epididymitis Inclusion conjunctivitis Listeriosis LRTI Lymphogranuloma venereum Plague Psittacosis Q Fever Rickettsial disease Rocky Mountain Spotted Fever Rosacea Shigellosis Staphylococcal SSTIs Syphilis (PCN allergy) Tularemia Uncomplicated gonorrhea Urethritis URTI Vincent's infection *(Fusobacterium fusiforme)* Yaws
Non-FDA-Approved Indications	Lyme disease Malaria prophylaxis
Pharmacodynamics	Limited PD data, bacteriostatic, +/− PAE
Pharmacokinetics	Hepatic metabolism; renal excretion (except doxycycline—feces)

Antimicrobial	Tetracyclines
Distribution	Body fluids—readily Bone—readily CSF—minimal/poor (↑ with inflamed meninges) Placenta—crosses Tissues—readily
Adverse Effects	Black tongue syndrome (benign; usually reversible on discontinuation) Contraindicated in children (due to tooth discoloration and inhibition of bone growth) and CrCl <10 mL/min (due to accumulation) Esophageal ulceration and/or esophagitis Fatty liver syndrome (mainly with IV tetracycline) GI Increased LFTs Phototoxicity Vestibular toxicity (minocycline)
Drug Interactions	Acitretin Chelation with mutivalent cations Decreased efficacy of estrogen Increased digoxin levels Isotretinoin Methotrexate
Monitoring	LFTs with prolonged therapy
Resistance Mechanisms	Efflux pumps (tet[B]) Ribosomal protection proteins
Comments	Doxycycline preferred in patients with renal failure Minocycline has better activity against CA-MRSA Minocycline is more lipophilic than tetracycline and may improve penetration into parasitic cells Not used for severe intra-abdominal infections or UTIs

III.3 ANTIVIRALS

III.3.1   ANTIVIRAL AGENTS FOR HSV, CMV, AND VZV

Antiviral	Acyclovir	Cidofovir	Famciclovir	Foscarnet	Ganciclovir	Valacyclovir	Valganciclovir
Trade Name	Zovirax	Vistide	Famvir	Foscavir	Cytovene-IV	Valtrex	Valcyte
Mechanism of Action	Inhibits viral DNA synthesis	Suppresses CMV replication by selective inhibition of viral DNA synthesis	Inhibits viral DNA synthesis	Inhibits viral RNA and DNA polymerases	Inhibits viral DNA synthesis	Inhibits viral DNA synthesis	Inhibits viral DNA synthesis
Spectrum of Activity Summary	HSV CMV (unlabeled use)	CMV	HSV	CMV HSV	CMV HSV	HSV VZV CMV (unlabeled)	CMV HSV
FDA-Approved Indications	• Genital HSV • HSV encephalitis	Treatment of CMV retinitis in patients with AIDS	• Treatment of HSV • Treatment and suppression of genital herpes • Treatment of herpes labialis	• Treatment of acyclovir-resistant HSV infections in immunocompromised patients • Treatment of CMV retinitis in patients with AIDS	Treatment of CMV retinitis	• Treatment of HSV • Treatment of genital herpes • Treatment of herpes labialis • Chickenpox in children	• Treatment of CMV retinitis in AIDS patients • Prevention of CMV in high-risk patients
Non-FDA-Approved Indications	• Prevention of HSV re-activation			CMV prophylaxis for cancer patients		Prophylaxis of HSV, VZV, and CMV infections	

Non-FDA-Approved Indications (*Cont'd*)	• Prevention of VZV • Treatment and prevention of recurrent mucosal and cutaneous HSV infections						
Elimination	Renal	Renal	Renal	Renal	Renal	Renal	Renal
Adverse Effects	• Diarrhea • Headache • Malaise • Nausea • Vomiting	Black box warnings: • Nephrotoxicity • Neutropenia CNS: headache, fever, chills, pain Dermatologic: alopecia, rash GI: nausea, vomiting, diarrhea Heme: anemia, neutropenia Neuromuscular: weakness Ocular: uveitis Renal: increased SCr, proteinuria	• Diarrhea • Fatigue • Headache • Nausea	Black box warnings: • Nephrotoxicity • Seizures Electrolyte abnormalities (Ca, PO_4, Mg, K), anemia	Boxed warning: • Neutropenia • Anemia • Thrombocytopenia • Anorexia • Diarrhea • Fever • Increased SCr • Vomiting	• Abdominal pain • Headache • Increased ALT and AST • Nasopharyngitis • Nausea • Neutropenia	Boxed warnings: • Neutropenia, anemia, thrombocytopenia • Anorexia • Diarrhea • Fever • Headache • Hypertension • Increased SCr • Vomiting

(continued)

Antiviral	Acyclovir	Cidofovir	Famciclovir	Foscarnet	Ganciclovir	Valacyclovir	Valganciclovir
Drug Interactions	• Avoid with the Zoster vaccine • May increase levels of mycophenolate, tenofivir, zidovudine	Cidofovir may increase the levels of tenofovir	Avoid with the Zoster vaccine	If possible, avoid use with: acyclovir-valacyclovir; AMGs; amphotericin B; cyclosporine; methotrexate; tacrolimus	• Avoid concomitant use with imipenem/cilastatin; may result in CNS toxicity (seizures); avoid if possible • May increase levels of mycophenolate, tenofivir, NRTIs	• Avoid with the Zoster vaccine • May increase levels of mycophenolate, tenofivir, zidovudine	• Concomitant use with imipenem/cilastatin may result in CNS toxicity (seizures); avoid if possible • May increase levels of mycophenolate, tenofivir, NRTIs
Dose	• 200 mg Q4h (5 times a day) or 400 mg TID (800 mg Q4h for shingles) • CrCl 10–25 mL/min = 800 mg Q8h (if going to give 800 mg Q4h dose) • CrCl ≤10 mL/min = 200 mg Q12h (800 mg Q12h [if going to give 800 mg Q4h dose])	5 mg/kg IV every week × 2, then 5 mg/kg IV every other week × 14–21 days	• 500 mg Q8h • CrCl 40–59 mL/min = 500 mg Q12h • CrCl 20–39 mL/min = 500 mg Q24h • CrCl <20 mL/min = 250 mg Q24h • HD = 250 mg as single dose post-dialysis session	60 mg/kg IV every 8h or 90 mg/kg IV every 12h × 14–21 days, then 90–120 mg/kg IV every 24h	Induction: • CrCl >50–69 mL/min = 2.5 mg/kg/dose Q12h • CrCl 25–49 mL/min = 2.5 mg/kg/dose Q24h • CrCl 10–24 mL/min = 1.25 mg/kg/dose Q24h	• 1 g TID • CrCl 30–49 mL/min = 1 g Q12h • CrCl 10–29 mL/min = 1 g Q24h • CrCl <10 mL/min= 500 mg Q24h • HD = dose post-dialysis	CMV retinitis: Induction: 900 mg BID × 21 days Maintenance: 900 mg daily HD: Not recommended; ganciclovir should be used. Prevention following transplant: 900 mg daily

	Dose (Cont'd)	**Monitoring**
	• HD = dose post-dialysis	• BUN • CBC • Liver enzymes • SCr • Urinalysis
		• Serum creatinine • Urine protein • WBC
		• CBC (long-term use only)
		• Electrolytes • CBC • SCr
	• CrCl <10 mL/min = 1.25 mg/kg/dose TIW following dialysis Maintenance: • CrCl >50–69 mL/min = 2.5 mg/kg/dose Q24h • CrCl 25–49 mL/min = 1.25 mg/kg/dose Q24h • CrCl 10–24 mL/min = 0.625 mg/kg/dose Q24h • CrCl <10 mL/min = 0.625 mg/kg/dose TIW following dialysis	• CBC with differential • Platelets • SCr
	Induction: • CrCl 40–59 mL/min = 450 mg BID • CrCl 25–39 mL/min = 450 mg daily • CrCl 10–24 mL/min = 450 mg every 2 days Maintenance: • CrCl 40–59 mL/min = 450 mg daily • CrCl 25–39 mL/min = 450 mg every 2 days • CrCl 10–24 mL/min = 450 mg twice weekly	• CBC • Platelets • Retinal exam (at least every 4–6 weeks) • SCr

(continued)

Antiviral	Acyclovir	Cidofovir	Famciclovir	Foscarnet	Ganciclovir	Valacyclovir	Valganciclovir
Resistance Mechanisms	Alterations in thymidine kinase and/or DNA polymerase	Point mutations in DNA polymerase	Alterations in thymidine kinase and/or DNA polymerase	Point mutations in DNA polymerase	Point mutations in DNA polymerase	Alterations in thymidine kinase and/or DNA polymerase	Point mutations in DNA polymerase
Comments	Dosing should be based on ideal body weight. Low oral bioavailability (15–20%). IV formulation may be nephrotoxic—administer with fluids. Resistance uncommon in immunocompetent patients	Probenecid must be administered with each dose of cidofovir. HSV resistant to acyclovir due to thymidine kinase mutations typically remain susceptible to cidofovir (do not require activation for intracellular activity) unless concomitant DNA polymerase mutations. May retain susceptibity in some foscarnet-resistant viral strains		Adequate hydration is essential to mitigating the nephrotoxicity of foscarnet (1 L with each dose). HSV resistant to acyclovir due to thymidine kinase mutations typically remain susceptible to foscarnet (do not require activation for intracellular activity) unless concomitant DNA polymerase mutations	Carcinogenic and teratogenic effects in animal studies. Females should use contraception and males should use barrier method for at least 90 days post therapy. Hazardous agent: Use PPE	Higher oral bioavailability than acyclovir (55–70%)	PPE should be used when handling the drug

III.3.2   ANTIVIRAL AGENTS FOR INFLUENZA

Antiviral	Amantadine	Oseltamivir	Peramivir	Rimantadine	Zanamivir
Trade Name	N/A	Tamiflu	Papivab	Flumadine	Relenza
Mechanism of Action	Inhibits viral DNA synthesis	Inhibits influenza virus neuraminidase, enzyme-altering virus release	Inhibits influenza virus neuraminidase, enzyme-altering virus release	Inhibits viral DNA synthesis	Inhibits influenza virus neuraminidase, enzyme-altering virus release
Spectrum of Activity Summary	Influenza A	Influenza A and B	Influenza A and B	Influenza A	Influenza A and B
FDA-Approved Indications	• Prophylaxis and treatment of influenza A (no longer recommended due to resistance issues) • Treatment of parkinsonism • Treatment of drug-induced EPS	• Treatment of uncomplicated acute illness caused by influenza A or B who have been symptomatic for less than 2 days • Prophylaxis against influenza A or B infection	• Treatment of uncomplicated, acute illness caused by influenza A or B who have been symptomatic for less than 2 days	• Prophylaxis (adults and children > 1 yo) and treatment (adults) of influenza A infection	• Treatment of uncomplicated acute illness caused by influenza A or B who have been symptomatic for less than 2 days • Prophylaxis against influenza A or B infection
Elimination	Renal	Renal	Renal	Renal	Renal
Adverse Effects	CNS: agitation, anxiety, ataxia, confusion, dizziness CV: orthostatic hypotension, peripheral edema Dermatological: livedo reticularis	GI: vomiting, nausea, abdominal pain, diarrhea Ocular: conjunctivitis Respiratory: epistaxis	CNS: insomnia, hallucinations, delirium Hematologic: neutropenia Neuromuscular: Increased CPK GI: diarrhea	CNS: insomnia, impaired concentration, dizziness, nervousness GI: nausea, anorexia, vomiting, xerostomia, abdominal pain	CNS: headache GI: throat/tonsil discomfort/pain Respiratory: nasal signs and symptoms, cough

(continued)

Antiviral	Amantadine	Oseltamivir	Peramivir	Rimantadine	Zanamivir
Adverse Effects (*Cont'd*)	GI: anorexia, nausea, constipation, diarrhea, xerostomia Respiratory: dry nose		Endocrine: increasd serum glucose	Neuromuscular and skeletal: weakness	
Drug Interactions	• Amantadine may increase the levels of: trimethoprim • Amantadine may decrease the levels of: typical antipsychotics, influenza virus vaccine (live/attenuated) • Atypical antipsychotics and metoclopramide may decrease amantadine levels	• Levels of oseltamivir may be increased by probenecid • Oseltamivir may decrease the levels/effects of influenza virus vaccine (live/attenuated)	• Peramivir may decrease the levels of: influenza virus vaccine (live/attenuated)	• MAO inhibitors may increase levels of rimantadine • Rimantadine may decrease the levels/effects of influenza virus vaccine (live/attenuated)	Zanamivir may decrease levels/effect of: influenza virus/vaccine (live/attenuated)
Dose	Influenza A treatment: 200 mg daily or 100 mg BID (initiate within 24–48 hrs after onset of symptoms) Influenza A prophylaxis: 200 mg daily or 100 mg BID (BID dosing for treatment or prophylaxis may decrease CNS effects)	Treatment: to be initiated within 48 hours of symptoms Prophylaxis: 75 mg daily CrCl 10–30 mL/min = 75 mg QOD or 30 mg daily Treatment: 75 mg BID × 5 days (may consider 150 PO BID if severe influenza [virulent strain, B strain])	Influenza A treatment: 600 mg daily as a single dose CrCl 30–49 mL/min = 200 mg IV as a single dose CrCl 10–29 mL/min = 100 mg IV as a single dose	Influenza A Prophylaxis: 100 mg BID (elderly: 100 mg daily) Treatment: 100 mg BID (elderly: 100 mg daily) CrCl>30 mL/min = dose adjustment not required CrCl<30 mL/min = 100 mg daily	Prophylaxis: 2 inhalations (10 mg) daily for 10 days (household setting) Prophylaxis: 2 inhalations (10 mg) daily for 28 days (community outbreak) Treatment: 2 inhalations (10 mg) BID for 5 days

			Severe hepatic dysfunction: 100 mg daily
Dose (Cont'd)	Drug-induced EPS: 100 mg BID; up to 300 mg/day in divided doses Hemodialysis: 200 mg every 7 days Parkinson's disease: 100 mg BID as monotherapy; may increase to 400 mg/day in divided doses, if necessary. Start at 100 mg daily if giving other anti-parkinson drugs CrCl 30–50 mL/min = 200 mg on day 1 then 100 mg daily CrCl 15–29 mL/min = 200 mg on day 1 then 100 mg on alternate days CrCl <15 mL/min = 200 mg every 7 days	Prophylaxis: 75 mg QOD or 30 mg daily HD: 30 mg after every other session CAPD: 30 mg once weekly	ESRD requiring HD = 100 mg IV as a single dose, given after dialysis	
Monitoring	Renal function BP	Mental status changes	Renal function Rash	GI and CNS effects, especially in elderly or patients with renal or hepatic impairment

(continued)

Antiviral	Amantadine	Oseltamivir	Peramivir	Rimantadine	Zanamivir
Resistance Mechanisms	Low genetic barrier for resistance; single mutation in the target viral protein (M_2)	Mutations in neuraminidase or viral protein hemagglutinin active sites	Presumed mutations in neuraminidase or viral protein hemagglutinin active sites	Low genetic barrier for resistance; single mutation in the target viral protein (M_2)	Mutations in neuraminidase or viral protein hemagglutinin active sites Peramivir Presumed mutations in neuraminidase or viral protein hemagglutinin active sites
Comments	Due to resistance issues, amantadine is no longer recommended for prophylaxis of influenza A. Those with severe CNS effects may respond better to rimantadine.	Take with food to improve tolerance Cross-resistance with zanamivir	Rare cases of serious skin reactions, including Stevens-Johnson syndrome and erythema mutiforme have occurred	Cross-resistance with amantadine	Zanamivir powder should never be given via nebulizer for ventilated patients (clogs ET tube) Cross-resistance with oseltamivir

PART IV

What Patient- or Disease State-Specific Factors Affect Your Decision?

IV.1   β-LACTAM ALLERGIES AND CROSS-REACTIVITY

Penicillin (PCN) is the most frequently reported cause of drug allergy. Up to 5–10% of the general population report PCN allergy however, approximately 95% of patients who report allergy are not truly allergic.[1-6] Beta-lactam cross-allergy is an area of debate and is attributable to similarities in the side chains between PCN and other beta-lactams. Historically, rates of cross-reactivity were reported to be up to 10% for cephalosporins and 40% for carbapenems. Newer literature suggests <3% and <1% rates of cross-reactivity for cephalosporins and carbapenems, respectively, and no chance of cross-reactivity to monobactams.[7-14] Allergies lead to the use of less efficacious and more toxic antimicrobials that may also have a higher risk of resistance development.

TYPES OF ALLERGIC REACTIONS[15]

The four types of allergic reactions are described below:[15]
- **Type I***—Immediate in onset (usually within one hour of exposure) and mediated by IgE and mast cells and/or basophils
  - Caused by specific antibodies to the drug
  - Most common signs/symptoms: urticaria, angioedema, anaphylaxis, or anaphylactic shock
- **Type II**—Delayed in onset (usually >72 hours) and caused by antibody (usually IgG)- mediated cell destruction
  - E.g., transfusion reactions including hemolytic anemia
- **Type III**—Delayed in onset (>72 hours, but up to 10 to 21 days) and caused by IgG:drug immune complex deposition and complement activation
  - E.g., serum sickness, Stevens Johnson syndrome
- **Type IV***—Delayed in onset (>72 hours) and T-cell mediated
  - E.g., maculopapular rash, contact dermatitis

*Drug allergies are most commonly associated with Types I and IV.

β-LACTAM ALLERGY CLARIFICATION QUESTIONS

In light of β-lactam allergy over-reporting combined with limited new antimicrobial treatment options, careful allergy assessment should be performed by asking clarifying questions when PCN (or other β-lactam) allergies are reported. This can easily be incorporated into the medication history and reconciliation process to assist with interpretation of the true allergy potential. All pertinent information should be thoroughly documented in the medical record.

Clarification Questions	Purpose	Comments
What specific drug caused the allergic reaction?	Determines the exact causative agent and helps to identify possible alternatives	• Oftentimes allergies are reported as vague drug class allergies as opposed to a specific agent within the class (e.g., PCN versus dicloxacillin or amoxicillin, etc.) • It is helpful to provide the patient with a short list of examples to help remember the exact name of the drug ◦ Offer both generic and brand names and oral and IV options

Clarification Questions	Purpose	Comments
What dosage form of this agent was utilized when the reaction occurred?	May determine the onset of allergic reaction symptoms	• IM/IV administration may have more rapid symptom onset, whereas the oral formulation may be delayed due to absorption time
What allergic reaction-associated symptoms were experienced at the time of the reaction?	Determines likelihood of true allergy and provides information on the reaction severity	• Severe reaction symptoms: urticaria, laryngeal edema, angioedema, wheezing, signs/symptoms of cardiorespiratory collapse, etc. ○ Maculopapular rashes are more consistent with an IgG-mediated reaction and do not always preclude re-challenge ○ Important to differentiate between pain, redness, or swelling at the injection site (i.e., injection site reaction versus allergic reaction, etc.) • Symptoms consistent with adverse effects rather than allergy: nausea, vomiting, diarrhea, headache, etc. • Unknown reaction: If unknown historic reaction, assess how long ago the reaction occurred and for subsequent receipt of other β-lactams without evidence of allergic reaction
How long after receiving the medication did the reaction occur?	May determine the type of reaction	• IgE-mediated reactions are usually immediate and generally occur within minutes to an hour; time of onset may be prolonged with the oral formulation • If a severe reaction (not rash/pruritus) developed more than 6 hours after receiving the β-lactam, consider alternative cause of symptoms
What medical therapy was required to manage the reaction?	Provides information on the reaction severity	• Observation • Medications: epinephrine, diphenhydramine, steroids, etc. • ED visit, hospitalization, ICU admission (+/− mechanical ventilation), or physician visit
Who observed or helped identify or confirm the reaction as an allergy?	Validates the likelihood of a true allergy	• Was the allergy witnessed by a nurse, physician, pharmacist, parent/guardian, etc. • If available, review provider/nursing notes at the time of exposure for confirmation
How long ago did the reaction occur? Was the reaction greater than or less than 10 years ago?	Determines the likelihood of current allergy potential	• IgE antibodies to PCN wane over time (validated with PCN skin testing and observational studies) ○ Patients who have experienced a true allergic reaction at a young age may tolerate later in life • After 10 years, 80% of patients with a PCN allergy have been shown to lose their sensitivity reaction to PCN and will often not experience the same reaction upon re-challenge

Clarification Questions	Purpose	Comments
What other antimicrobials has the patient received after the reaction occurred? If patient has received other β-lactams, assess which agents and determine if any similar symptoms were experienced.	Determine the safety of agents that have cross-reactivity potential	• If a patient has subsequently tolerated other β-lactams, these agents can be utilized

AGENTS WITH SIMILAR SIDE CHAINS[16,17]

Antimicrobial	Antimicrobials with Similar R1 Side Chains That Are Likely to Cross-React
Penicillins (ampicillin/amoxicillin)	First-generation cephalosporins: • Cefadroxil • Cephalexin Second-generation cephalosporins: • Cefaclor • Cefprozil
Ceftazidime	Aztreonam

RECOMMENDATION[18]

In patients with a documented IgE-mediated reaction to penicillin:

- Third- and fourth-generation cephalosporins may be safely administered
- Avoid first- and second-generation cephalosporins with side chains similar to that of penicillin (i.e., cefaclor, cefadroxil, cefprozil, and cephalexin)
- First- and second-generation cephalosporins with different side chains may be administered (i.e., cefazolin)
  - Cefazolin has a unique side chain that is different than any other β-lactam[19]
- Carbapenems may be used as likelihood of cross-reactivity is low

In patients with a documented IgE-mediated reaction to either aztreonam or ceftazidime, avoid both agents as they share the same side chain.

CONCLUSION

β-lactam allergies are considerably over-reported and lead to suboptimal antimicrobial utilization. Critical assessment and evaluation of patient allergies can be challenging; however with careful review of allergy history during the medication history and reconciliation process, certain β-lactams may be safely utilized.

REFERENCES

1. Allergic reactions to long-term benzathine penicillin prophylaxis for rheumatic fever. International rheumatic fever study group. *Lancet.* 1991;337:1308–10.
2. Solensky R. Allergy to beta-lactam antibiotics. *J Allergy Clin Immunol.* 2012;130;1442–2.e5.
3. Wong BBL, Keith PK, Waserman S. Clinical history as a predictor of penicillin skin test outcome. *Ann Allergy Asthma Immunol.* 2006;97:169–74.
4. Borch JE, Anderson KE, Bindslev-Jensen C. The prevalence of suspected and challenge-verified penicillin allergy in a university hospital population. *Basic Clin Pharmacol Toxicol.* 2006;98:357–62.
5. Macy E, Schatz M, Lin C, et al. The falling rate of positive penicillin skin tests from 1995–2007. *Perm J.* 2009;13:12–18.
6. Frumin J, Gallagher JC. Allergic cross-sensitivity between penicillin, carbapenem, and monobactam antibiotics: what are the chances? *Ann Pharmacother.* 2009;43:304–15.
7. Novalbos A, Sastre J, Cuesta J, et al. Lack of allergic cross-reactivity to cephalosporins among patients allergic to penicillins. *Clin Exp Allergy.* 2001;31:438–43.
8. Apter AJ, Kinman JL, Bilker WB, et al. Is there cross-reactivity between penicillins and cephalosporins? *Am J Med.* 2006;119:354.e11–9.
9. Phillips E, Knowles SR, Weber EA, et al. Cephalexin tolerated despite delayed aminopenicillin reactions. *Allergy.* 2001;56:790.
10. Goodman EJ, Morgan MJ, Johnson PA, et al. Cephalosporins can be given to penicillin-allergic patients who do not exhibit an anaphylactic response. *J Clin Anesth.* 2001;13:561–64.
11. Daulat S, Solensky R, Earl HS, et al. Safety of cephalosporin administration to patients with histories of penicillin allergy. *J Allergy Clin Immunol.* 2004;113:1220–22.
12. Ahmed KA, Fox SJ, Frigas E, et al. Clinical outcome in the use of cephalosporins in pediatric patients with a history of penicillin allergy. *Int Arch Allergy Immunol.* 2012;158:405–10.
13. Park MA, Koch CA, Klemawesch P, et al. Increased adverse drug reactions to cephalosporins in penicillin allergy patients with positive penicillin skin test. *Int Arch Allergy Immunol.* 2010;153:268–73.
14. Romano A, Gaeta F, Valluzzi RL, et al. IgE-mediated hypersensitivity to cephalosporins: cross-reactivity and tolerability of penicillins, monobactams, and carbapenems. *J Allergy Clin Immunol.* 2010;126:994–9.
15. Chang C, Mahmood MM, Teuber SS, et al. Overview of penicillin allergy. *Clin Rev Allergy Immunol.* 2012;43:84–97.
16. Miranda A, Blanca M, Vega JM, et al. Cross-reactivity between a penicillin and a cephalosporin with the same side chain. *J Allergy Clin Immunol.* 1996;98:671–7.
17. Sastre J, Quijano LD, Novalbos A, et al. Clinical cross-reactivity between amoxicillin and cephadroxil in patients allergic to amoxicillin and with good tolerance of penicillin. *Allergy.* 1996;51:383–6.
8. Campagna JD, Bond MC, Schabelman E, et al. The use of cephalosporins in penicillin-allergic patients: a literature review. *J Emerg Med.* 2012;42:612–20.
9. Benninger MS. Cephalosporin use in treatment of patients with penicillin allergies. *J Am Pharm Assoc.* 2008;48:530.

IV.2   ADULT RENAL DOSING CHART

Generic Name	IV	PO	Dose Range	Interval (Based on Creatinine Clearance)		
				>50 mL/min	10–50 mL/min	<10 mL/min
Acyclovir	X	X	IV: 5–10 mg/kg/dose **Use IBW if obese** PO: 200–800 mg	IV: Q8h PO: 3–5 times a day	IV: Q12h PO: Q8h	IV: Q24h PO: Q12h
Amantadine		X	100–200 mg	100 mg BID or 200 mg Q24h	30–50 mL/min: 200 mg on day 1 then 100 mg Q24h / 15–29 mL/min: 200 mg on day 1 then 100 mg on alternate days	200 mg every 7 days
Amikacin	X		Traditional: 5–7.5 mg/kg/dose / Extended Interval: 15–20 mg/kg	See Aminoglycoside Pharmacokinetic Chart for details		
Amoxicillin		X	500 mg	Q8h		Q24h
			875 mg		>30 mL/min: 250–500 mg Q12h / 10–30 mL/min: 250–500 mg Q24h	Not recommended
Amoxicillin/ clavulanate		X	500 mg	Q8h		Q24h
			875 mg	Q12h	>30 mL/min: Q8h / 10–30 mL/min: Q12h	Not recommended
Amphotericin B (conventional)	X		0.4–1 mg/kg/dose	Q24h	Q24h	Q24h
Amphotericin B Lipid Complex (Abelcet)	X		5 mg/kg/dose	Q24h	Q24h	Q24h
Amphotericin B				Q24h	Q24h	Q24h

Drug			Dose			
Ampicillin	X	X	IV: 1–2 g / PO: 250–500 mg	Q6h	Q8h	Q12h
Ampicillin/sulbactam	X		3 g	Q6h	31–50 mL/min: Q8h; 11–30 mL/min: Q12h	Q24h
Anidulafungin	X		100–200 mg	200 mg on day 1 then 100 mg Q24h	No adjustment for renal dysfunction	
Azithromycin	X	X	500 mg	Q24h	No adjustment for renal dysfunction	
Aztreonam	X	X	1–2 g	Q8h	31–50 mL/min: Q8h; 11–30 mL/min: Q12h	Q24h
Caspofungin	X		50–70 mg	70 mg on day 1 then 50 mg Q24h	No adjustment for renal dysfunction	
Cefaclor	X		500 mg	Q8h	500 mg Q12h	250 mg Q12h
Cefadroxil	X		500 mg	Q12h	25–50 mL/min: Q12h; 10–25 mL/min: Q24h	Q36h
Cefazolin	X		1–2 g	Q8h	Q12h	Q24h
Cefdinir	X	X	600 mg	Q24h	300 mg Q12h for CAP, 600 mg Q24h for other infections; 300 mg Q24h for CrCl < 30 mL/min	
Cefditoren	X		200–400 mg	Q12h	30–49 mL/min: 200 mg Q12h; <30 mL/min: 200 mg Q24h	200 mg Q24h
Cefepime	X		Febrile neutropenia, Pseudomonas infection; 1–2 g	Q12h (CrCl >60 mL/min) / Q8h (CrCl >60 mL/min)	Q24h (CrCl <60 mL/min); Q12h (CrCl 30–60 mL/min); Q24h (CrCl < 30 mL/min)	
Cefixime	X		400 mg	Q24h	260 mg Q24h	200 mg Q24h
Cefotaxime	X	X	1–2 g	Q6–8h	Q8–12h	Q24h
Cefotetan	X		1–2 g	Q12h	31–50 mL/min: Q12h; 10–29 mL/min: Q24h	Q48h

(continued)

Generic Name	IV	PO	Dose Range	Interval (Based on Creatinine Clearance)			
				>50 mL/min	10–50 mL/min		<10 mL/min
					31–50 mL/min	10–29 mL/min	
Cefoxitin	X		1–2 g	Q6h	Q6h	Q8–12h	Q24h
Cefpodoxime		X	100–400 mg	Q12h	Q12h	Q24h	Q24h
Cefprozil		X	250–500 mg	Q12h	Q12h	Q24h	Q24h
Ceftaroline	X		600 mg	Q12h Q8h (>100 kg and BMI > 40)	400 mg Q12h 600 mg Q12h	300 mg Q12h 400 mg Q12h	200 mg Q12h 300 mg Q12h
Ceftazidime	X		1–2 g	Q8h	Q12h	Q24h	Q24h
Ceftazidime/avibactam	X		2.5 g	Q8h	1.25 g Q8h	0.94 g Q12h	0.94 g Q24h
Ceftolazane/tazobactam	X		1.5 g	Q8h	750 mg Q8h	375 mg Q12h	750 mg × 1 then 150 mg Q8h
Ceftibuten		X	400 mg	Q24h	200 mg Q24h	100 mg Q24h	100 mg Q24h
Ceftriaxone	X		1–2 g	Q24h (Q12h for meningitis)	No adjustment for renal dysfunction		
Cefuroxime	X	X	IV: 1.5 g PO: 500 mg	Q6h Q12h	Q12h		Q24h
Cephalexin		X	500 mg	Q6h	Q8h		Q12h

Drug	IV	PO	Dose	>30 mL/min	<30 mL/min
Cidofovir	X		5 mg/kg/dose	Induction: once weekly; Maintenance: every other week	Use not recommended
Ciprofloxacin	X	X	IV: 200–400 mg; PO: 250–750 mg (400 mg IV = 500 mg PO)	Q12h	Q24h
Clarithromycin		X	500 mg	Q12h	250 mg Q12h
Clindamycin	X	X	IV: 600–900 mg; PO: 300–450 mg	IV: Q8h; PO: Q6–8h	No dosage adjustment for renal dysfunction
Colistin	X		1–2.5 mg/kg/dose	>80 mL/min: 2.5 mg/kg Q12h; 40–79 mL/min: 1.25–1.9 mg/kg Q12h	25–39 mL/min: 1.25 mg/kg Q24h; 10–24 mL/min: 1.5 mg/kg Q36h; 1.5 mg/kg Q48h
Dalbavancin	X		500–1,000 mg	1000 mg × 1, followed by 500 mg × 1 one week later	750 mg × 1, followed by 375 mg × 1 one week later
Daptomycin	X		4 or 6 mg/kg/dose off-label 8–10 mg/kg/dose	>30 mL/min: Q24h	<30 mL/min: Q48h
Dicloxacillin		X	500 mg	Q6h	No dosage adjustment for renal dysfunction
Doripenem	X		500 mg	Q8h; 30–50 mL/min: 250 mg Q8h	11–29 mL/min: 250 mg Q12h; 250 mg Q24h
Doxycycline	X	X	100–200 mg	Q12h	No dosage adjustment for renal dysfunction
Ertapenem	X		1 g	>30 mL/min: 1 g Q24h	<30 mL/min: 500 mg Q24h
Erythromycin	X	X	500 mg	QID	No dosage adjustment for renal dysfunction

(continued)

Generic Name	IV	PO	Dose Range	Interval (Based on Creatinine Clearance) >50 mL/min	10–50 mL/min	<10 mL/min
Famciclovir		X	250–500 mg	(>60 mL/min) Q8h	(40–59 mL/min) 500 mg Q12h; (20–39 mL/min) 500 mg Q24h	(<20 mL/min) 250 mg Q24h
Fluconazole	X	X	100–1,200 mg	Q24h	200–400 mg Q24h	200–400 mg Q24h
Flucytosine		X	50–150 mg/kg/day	Q6h	37.5 mg Q12–24h; 37.5 mg Q24h	37.5 mg Q24–48h
Ganciclovir	X		Induction (I): 5 mg/kg/dose; Maintenance (M): 5 mg/kg/dose	(>70 mL/min) I: 5 mg/kg Q12h, M: 5 mg/kg Q24h; (50–69 mL/min) I: 2.5 mg/kg Q12h, M: 2.5 mg/kg Q24h	(25–49 mL/min) I: 2.5 mg/kg Q24h, M: 1.25 mg/kg Q24h; (10–24 mL/min) I: 1.25 mg/kg Q24h, M: 0.625 mg/kg Q24h	(<10 mL/min) I: 1.25 mg/kg 3 times/week, M: 0.625 mg/kg 3 times/week
Gentamicin	X		Traditional: 1–2.5 mg/kg/dose; Extended Interval: 4–7 mg/kg	See Aminoglycoside Pharmacokinetic Chart for details		
Imipenem/cilastatin	X		500–1,000 mg	Q6h	250–500 mg Q8h	250–500 mg Q12h
Itraconazole		X	200 mg	Loading dose of 200 mg Q8h × 3 days then maintenance dose of 200 mg Q12h	No dosage adjustment for renal dysfunction	
Ketoconazole		X	200–400 mg	Q24h	No dosage adjustment for renal dysfunction	
Levofloxacin	X	X	500–750 mg (250 mg may be used)	750 mg Q24h	750 mg Q48h	750 mg × 1, then 500 mg Q48h
Linezolid	X	X	600 mg	Q12h	No dosage adjustment for renal dysfunction	

			Standard	>51 mL/min	26–50 mL/min	10–25 mL/min	<10 mL/min
Meropenem	X		Standard	1 g Q8h	1 g Q12h	500 mg Q12h	500 mg Q24h
			Meningitis	2 g Q8h	2 g Q12h	1 g Q12h	1 g Q24h
Metronidazole	X	X	500 mg	Q8h	No dosage adjustment for renal dysfunction		
Micafungin	X		50–150 mg	Q24h	No dosage adjustment for renal dysfunction		
Minocycline	X	X	100–200 mg	200 mg × 1, then 100 mg Q12h	No dosage adjustment for renal dysfunction		
Moxifloxacin	X	X	400 mg	Q24h	No dosage adjustment for renal dysfunction		
Nafcillin	X	X	1–2 g	Q4–6h	No dosage adjustment for renal dysfunction		
Nitrofurantoin		X	50–100 mg	Macrobid: Q12h Furadantin, Macrodantin: Q6h	Use not recommended		
Norfloxacin		X	400 mg	Q12h	<30 mL/min Q24h		
Ofloxacin		X	200–400 mg	Q12h	20–50 mL/min 200–400 mg Q24h		<20 mL/min 200 mg Q24h
Oseltamivir		X	75 mg	Treatment: Q12h Prophylaxis: Q24h	30–50 mL/min Treatment: 30 mg Q12h Prophylaxis: 30 mg Q24h	<30 mL/min Treatment: 30 mg Q24h Prophylaxis: 30 mg Q48h	No data
Oxacillin	X		1–2 g	Q4–6h	No dosage adjustment in renal dysfunction		
Penicillin G	X	X	1–4 mg	Q4–6h	Q6–12h		Q12h
Penicillin VK	X		500 mg	Q6h	No dosage adjustment for renal dysfunction		
Piperacillin		X	3–4 g	Q6h	30–50 mL/min Q8h	10–30 mL/min Q12h	Q12h

(continued)

Generic Name	IV	PO	Dose Range	Interval (Based on Creatinine Clearance)		
				>50 mL/min	10–50 mL/min	<10 mL/min
Piperacillin/tazobactam	X		3.375–4.5 g	Q6h	Q8h	Q12h
Posaconazole	X	X	Oral suspension: 200–400 mg; Oral tablets and IV: 300 mg Q12h day one then 300 mg once daily		Suspension: Q8h; Tablet/IV: Q12h on day 1, then Q24h; No dosage adjustment for renal dysfunction	
Quinupristin/dalfopristin	X		7.5 mg/kg/dose	Q8h	No dosage adjustment for renal dysfunction	
Rimantadine		X	100 mg	Q12h	<30 mL/min 100 mg Q24h	
Streptomycin	IM		1–2 g	Q12–24h	Q24–72h	Q72–96h
Sulfamethoxazole/trimethoprim	X	X	IV: 2.5–5 mg/kg/dose	Q6–8h	Q12h	Q24h
			PO: 800/160 mg	Q12h	Q12h	Q24h
Tedizolid	X	X	200 mg	Q24h	No dosage adjustment for renal dysfunction	
Telavancin	X		10 mg/kg/dose	Q24h	30–49 mL/min 7.5 mg/kg Q12h	<30 mL/min 10 mg/kg Q48h
Tetracycline		X	250–500 mg	>80 mL/min Q6h	50–79 mL/min Q8–12h; 10–49 mL/min Q12–24h	<10 mL/min Q24h
Telithromycin		X	800 mg	Q24h	<30 mL/min 600 mg Q24h	
Ticarcillin/clavulanate	X		3.1 g	Q6h	Q8h	Q12h

Drug		Dose	>60 mL/min	40–59 mL/min	25–39 mL/min	10–24 mL/min
Tigecycline	X	50 mg	100 mg loading dose × 1, then 50 mg Q12h	No dosage adjustment for renal dysfunction		
Tobramycin	X	Traditional: 1–2.5 mg/kg/dose; Extended Interval: 4–7 mg/kg	See Aminoglycoside Pharmacokinetic Chart for details			
Valacyclovir	X	1–2 g	Dose and frequency dependent upon indication; Renal dosage adjustment necessary			
Valganciclovir	X	450–900 mg	**I:** 900 mg Q12h **M:** 900 mg Q24 or 450 mg Q12h	**I:** 450 mg Q12h **M:** 450 mg Q24h	**I:** 450 mg Q24h **M:** 450 mg Q48h	**I:** 450 mg Q48h **M:** 450 mg twice weekly
Vancomycin	X	IV: 15–20 mg/kg/dose; PO: 125 mg	IV: See Vancomycin Dosing and Pharmacokinetics Chart			
			Q6h	Q6h	Q6h	Q6h
Voriconazole	X	IV: 6 mg/kg load Q12h × 2 followed by 4 mg/kg Q12h maintenance; PO: 200–300 mg Q12h (Varies by indication)	See prescribing indication for complete dosing information; If CrCl <50 mL/min, avoid IV voriconazole due to sulfobutylether cyclodextrin vehicle			
Zanamivir	INH	2 INH (10 mg total)	Q12h	No dosage adjustment for renal dysfunction		

IV.3 ANTIMICROBIAL PHARMACODYNAMICS

The figure below visually represents the pharmacodynamics of antimicrobials.

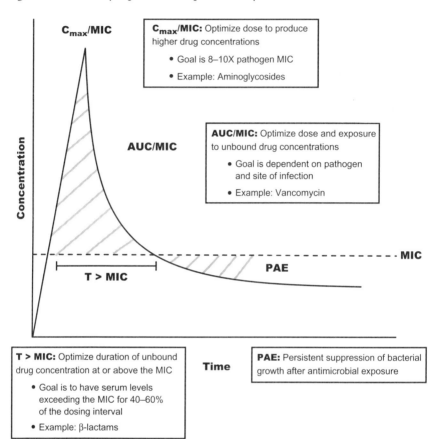

ANTIMICROBIAL PHARMACODYNAMICS

Parameter	Definition	Limitations

MIC (Minimum Inhibitory Concentration)	• Concentration at which a standard inoculum of 10^5 organisms are inhibited after 24–48 hours
	• Interpretation of MICs requires knowledge of:
	  ○ Pharmacokinetics of the drug in humans
	  ○ Success of a particular drug in eradicating bacteria at various body sites
	• Published by the Clinical Laboratory Standards Institute (CLSI or EUCAST)
	• Established by analysis of the following data:
	  ○ Microbiologic data
	  ○ Pharmacokinetic and pharmacodynamic data
	  ○ Clinical studies that compare MICs with microbiological eradication and clinical efficacy (occurs prior to FDA approval)
		• *In vitro* conditions differ from those at infection site
		• Only reflects a specific time point
		• *In vitro* drug concentrations remain constant
		• Measured against standard inoculum
		• Lacks information on:
		  ○ Rate of bactericidal activity
		  ○ Persistent effects
		• *In vitro* tests may not adequately predict outcome

MBC (Minimum Bactericidal Concentration)	• Concentration at which a 99.9% reduction in the standard inoculum occurs • Difficult to perform	
Breakpoint	• Published by the CLSI and set by the FDA upon drug approval process • Breakpoints determine susceptible, intermediate, and resistant • Should reflect the MIC_{90} and the serum level attained by the drug • When the sensitivity of bacteria surpasses a predetermined concentration of drug (breakpoint), the bacteria is said to be resistant • Breakpoint concentrations are specific to organism/drug combinations. As such, the lowest MIC on a susceptibility report does not always indicate the best therapeutic option	

CLSI Interpretation	• *Susceptible:* Infection due to the strain may be appropriately treated with that antimicrobial at recommended doses
	• *Susceptible Dose-Dependent:* Infection may be treated with that antimicrobial when higher doses or more frequent dosing intervals are utilized or both
	• *Intermediate:* A microorganism falls into a range of susceptibility in which the MIC approaches or exceeds the level of antimicrobial that can be achieved and for which clinical response is likely to be less than with a susceptible strain
	  – *Exceptions:*
	    ○ If an antimicrobial is highly concentrated in a body fluid such as urine
	    ○ If higher than normal doses can safely be administered, may consider the use of that drug
	• *Resistant:* Strains are not inhibited by the usually achievable systemic concentrations with normal dosage schedules	

Bacteriostatic	• <3 log kill at 18–24 hours after drug administration	
Bactericidal	• ≥3 log kill or 99.9% reduction in starting inoculums at 18–24 hours after drug administration	

IV.4   ANTIMICROBIAL PHARMACOKINETICS

IV.4.1   AMINOGLYCOSIDE PHARMACOKINETICS AND DOSING

Empiric Conventional Dosing

Step 1: Determine dosing weight

Male Ideal Body Weight (IBW) = 50 kg + 2.3(height >60 inches)
Female Ideal Body Weight (IBW) = 45.5 kg + 2.3(height >60 inches)

Patient Weight Status		Dosing Weight (kg)
Normal	IBW < ABW < 1.3(IBW)	IBW
Underweight	ABW < IBW	ABW
Overweight (obese)	ABW > 1.3(IBW)	aBW

ABW = actual body weight; aBW = adjusted body weight

Adjusted body weight (aBW) = IBW + 0.4(ABW − IBW)

Step 2: Calculate estimated creatinine clearance

Dosing Weight

$$\text{Estimated CrCl} = \frac{140 - \text{age} \times \text{IBW}^*}{72 \times \text{Scr}} \times 0.85 \text{ for females}$$

(If patient is >65 yo or malnourished and SCr is < 0.8 mg/dL, use 0.8 mg/dL)

*If a patient is >30% above IBW, use aBW
[aBW = 0.4(ABW − IBW) = IBW]
*If a patient's ABW < IBW, use ABW

Step 3: Determine appropriate population volume of distribution (Vd) estimate

Estimated Volume of Distribution (Vd)	Patient Population
0.55 L/kg	Premature neonates
0.45 L/kg	Full-term neonates
0.4 ± 0.1 L/kg	Infants (>4 weeks – 1 year)
0.35 ± 0.15 L/kg	Children (1–13 years)
0.3 ± 0.1 L/kg	Adolescents (13–18 years)
0.25–0.3 L/kg	General medicine adult patients
0.385–0.4 L/kg	Overhydrated/edematous*

*Potential reasons for increased Vd include heart failure, peritonitis, edema, ascites, pregnancy, cystic fibrosis, and neonates

Step 4: Determine goal peak and trough serum concentrations

Target Serum Level Ranges for Traditional Aminoglycoside Dosing

Infection Type/Severity		Gentamicin and Tobramycin Targets		Amikacin	
		Peaks (mcg/mL)	Troughs (mcg/mL)	Peaks (mcg/mL)	Troughs (mcg/mL)
Gram Negative	Severe to life-threatening	8–10	<2	25–30	<8
	Moderate to mild	6–8	<2	20–25	<6
	UTI	4–6	<2	15–20	<6
Gram positive (for synergy)		3–5*	<2	—	

* Serum peak concentration monitoring is usually not necessary when used for synergy; however, periodic trough levels are suggested to ensure no accumulation—especially in the elderly and those with renal dysfunction.

Step 5: Calculate dose

$\text{Dose} = \text{DW} \times \text{Vd} \times \text{P}$
DW = dosing weight; Vd = population volume of distribution estimate; P = desired peak
Typical empiric dosing = 2 mg/kg; typical synergistic dosing = 1 mg/kg

Step 6: Determine frequency based on estimated creatinine clearance

↳ genta / tobra Amikacin 7–8 mg/kg

Creatinine Clearance	Dosing Frequency
≥60 mL/min	Q8h
40–59 mL/min	Q12h
20–39 mL/min	Q24h
<20 mL/min	One dose followed by levels

Step 7: Monitor steady state serum peak and trough concentrations with the third dose in patients expected to receive ≥3 days of aminoglycoside therapy. Peak concentrations (C_{peak}) should be obtained 30 minutes after the infusion to allow for the distribution phase. Trough concentrations (C_{trough}) should be obtained within 30 minutes prior to the administered dose. Frequency of levels is generally every 3 to 5 days. More frequent monitoring of serum levels may be appropriate for patients with unstable renal function. Monitor serum creatinine at least every 3 days or daily in patients with unstable renal function.

Monitor	When to Obtain/Frequency
Trough	Initial: within 30 minutes prior to the third dose (steady state) Subsequent: at steady state with dose adjustments or Q3–5 days in patients expected to receive ≥3 days of aminoglycoside
Peak	Initial: 30 minutes after the end of the infusion of the third dose Subsequent: at steady state with dose adjustments or Q3–5 days in patients expected to receive ≥3 days of aminoglycoside
Serum creatinine	Stable renal function: minimum Q3 days Unstable renal function: daily

DOSE ADJUSTMENTS based on serum concentrations (Sawchuk-Zaske Method):

Step 1: Verify dose administration and sampling times are appropriate

Step 2: Calculate k_e and $t_{1/2}$:

$$k_e = \frac{\ln(C_{peak}/C_{trough})}{\tau - (t_{tr} + t' + t_{pk})}$$

$$t_{1/2} = \frac{0.693}{k_e}$$

τ = Dosing interval
t_{tr} = time in hours between when trough drawn and next dose given
t' = length of infusion in hours (e.g., 0.5 hr)
t_{pk} = time in hours between when infusion ended and peak drawn
$t_{1/2}$ = half life

Step 3: Calculate the true peak at the end of the infusion ($C_{max\text{-}ss}$):

$$C_{max\text{-}ss} = C_{peak\,measured} \times e^{ke \times t_{pk}}$$

Step 4: If the trough was drawn early, calculate the true trough ($C_{min\text{-}ss}$):

$$C_{min\text{-}ss} = C_{trough\,measured} \times e^{-ke \times t_{tr}}$$

Δt = time between measured, early trough (C_{trough}) and time of appropriately drawn trough ($C_{min\text{-}ss}$) (e.g., when the next dose was administered)

Step 5: Calculate patient specific Vd:

$$Vd = \frac{(K_0/t')(1 - e^{-ke \times t'})}{(k_e)[(C_{max\text{-}ss}) - (C_{min\text{-}ss}) - e^{-ke \times t'})]}$$

Divide Vd by patient weight to get L/kg

Step 6: If the serum peak and trough concentrations are within the desired ranges, continue the current dosing regimen. If the measured serum peak and trough concentrations are not in the desired ranges, then a new dosing regimen should be designed using calculated patient-specific pharmacokinetic parameters (**go to Step 7**).

Step 7: Calculate the new dosing interval (τ):

$$\tau = \frac{\ln(C_{max\text{-}D}/C_{min\text{-}D})}{k_e} + t'$$

$C_{max\text{-}D}$ = desired peak
$C_{min\text{-}D}$ = desired trough

Step 8: Calculate a new maintenance dose (K_0):

$$K_0 = \frac{(C_{max-D})(k_e)(V_d)(1-e^{-ke \times \tau})}{(1-e^{-ke \times t'})}$$

NOTE: (K_0) = mg/hour (e.g., X mg/1 hr infusion)

Step 9: Calculate the estimated peak (estC_{peak}) and estimated trough (estC_{trough}) concentrations at steady-state with the new dosing regimen:

$$estC_{peak} = \frac{(K_0)(1-e^{-ke \times t'})}{(k_e)(V_d)(t')(1-e^{-ke \times \tau})}$$

$$estC_{trough} = (estC_{peak})(e^{-ke \times (T-t')})$$

Subsequent Monitoring:
- Repeat serum peak and trough concentrations should be done with a new dosing regimen or repeated if a noted change in renal function is observed.
- Trough concentrations should be obtained every 5 to 7 days in patients with stable renal function and hemodynamic status to assess for drug accumulation and minimize the risk for nephrotoxicity and ototoxicity.

Extended-Interval Aminoglycoside Dosing
The extended interval method is intended to maximize the therapeutic efficacy through concentration-dependent bactericidal activity (goal peak: minimum inhibitory concentration [MIC] ratio ≥8–10) and utilize the post-antibiotic effect while minimizing toxicity through a drug free interval (serum concentrations <0.5 mcg/mL).

Patient Selection:
Avoid in pediatric patients (age <13 years), acute or chronic renal insufficiency/ESRD, mycobacterial infections, patients with altered volume of distribution (ascites, cirrhosis, pregnancy, severe burns, hemodynamic instability), and for gram-positive synergy (including endocarditis).

Initial Dose:
- Tobramycin/gentamicin—7 mg/kg (may use 5 mg/kg for UTI)
- Amikacin—15 mg/kg

Initial Frequency:

Creatinine Clearance	Dosing Frequency
≥60 mL/min	Q24h
40–59 mL/min	Q36h
20–39 mL/min	Q48h (use caution)
<20 mL/min	Not recommended

Monitoring:
- Obtain random level 6–14 hours after the start of the first dose.
- Dosage adjustments should be made according to the Hartford Nomogram (Figure 1).
- After evaluation of the initial serum level, repeat levels should be evaluated every 5–7 days or earlier if renal function changes.

Important Notes:
- Because the Hartford Nomogram was based on a dose of 7 mg/kg, if a lower dose is being used, the resultant level should be multiplied by a factor equal to 7 mg divided by the dose used. (Example: If a patient is receiving 6 mg/kg/day and the 12h post-dose level was 4 mcg/mL, you would multiply the level by 1.16 (7/6) to give a level of 4.6 mcg/mL. This adjusted level is the one you would plot on the Hartford Nomogram.)
- If the level falls on the line, choose the longer interval for administration.
- If the aminoglycoside level falls off the nomogram, traditional dosing should be used.
- If once daily dosing is utilized for patients with altered Vd, such as cystic fibrosis (initial dose 10 mg/kg) patients or for postpartum infections, consider obtaining two random levels (2-hours post infusion [$C_{1random}$] and 10-hours post infusion) and calculate k_e, C_{pk}, and C_{tr}.

$$k_e = \frac{\ln(C_{1random}/C_{2random})}{\tau - \Delta t}$$

$C_{peak} = C_{1random} \times e^{-ket1}$ (t1 = time in hours after end of infusion of first random level)

$C_{trough} = C_{2random} \times e^{-ket2}$ (t2 = time in hours after end of infusion of second random level)

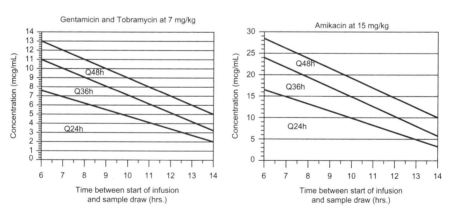

Figure 1   Hartford Nomograms

Source: Reproduced with permission from Nicolau DP, Freeman CD, Belliveau PP, et al. Experience with a once-daily aminoglycoside program administered to 2,184 adult patients. *Antimicrob Agents Chemother.* 1995;39(3):650–5.

Intermittent Dosing in End-Stage Renal Disease (ESRD)

Note that a variety of host- and dialysis-related factors affect the precise rate and quantity of drug removed. Therefore, monitoring of troughs (and peaks) is recommended. Unless a volume of distribution shift is expected, it may be adequate to remeasure only troughs to avoid drug accumulation.

Drugs	Indication	Dose and Frequency in Dialysis Patients	
		Hemodialysis	Peritoneal Dialysis
		Dose POST dialysis	Q48H, assumed
Gentamicin	Treatment, general	1.5–2 mg/kg	1.5–2 mg/kg
	Urinary Tract Infection	1 mg/kg	1 mg/kg
	Synergy	1 mg/kg	1 mg/kg
Tobramycin	Treatment, general	1.5–2 mg/kg	1.5–2 mg/kg
	Urinary Tract Infection	1 mg/kg	1 mg/kg
Amikacin	Treatment, general	7.5 mg/kg	7.5 mg/kg

Serum Trough Level:
- Serum trough levels should be performed pre-dialysis to *estimate post-dialysis* concentrations.
- It is estimated that ~50% is removed during high flux hemodialysis.

Hemodialysis:
- Target serum troughs (pre-dialysis) are usually 2–3 mcg/mL for gentamicin or tobramycin and 10–15 mcg/mL for amikacin.

Drug	Goal Post-Dialysis Trough Concentration (mcg/mL)
Gentamicin	<2
Tobramycin	<2
Amikacin	<6

Peritoneal Dialysis:
- The patient is considered a candidate for parenteral redosing when the serum trough level ("random") is <2 mcg/mL for gentamicin and <8 mcg/mL for amikacin. The doses empirically estimated may need to be adjusted.

Dosing in Continuous Renal Replacement Therapy (CRRT):
- Critically-ill patients receiving CRRT should be administered an initial dose (using the patient's calculated **Dosing Weight**) based on the indication for therapy.

Documented or Suspected Infection Due to:

Drug	Gram-Positive Bacteria (Synergy)	Gram-Negative Bacteria
Gentamicin	1 mg/kg	1.5–2 mg/kg
Tobramycin	—	1.5–2 mg/kg
Amikacin	—	5–7.5 mg/kg

Gram-Positive Synergy (Gentamicin):
- The initial dosing interval should be every 12 to 24 hours.
- A serum peak and trough concentration should be drawn with the 3rd or 4th dose to ensure clearance; peaks not usually necessary.

Documented or Suspected Gram-Negative Infection:
- Administer a one-time dose.
- *Random concentration* should be ordered at **24 hours** after loading dose administered.
- Subsequent doses should be determined using calculated, patient-specific pharmacokinetic parameters. *NOTE: ensure that CRRT was not interrupted between obtaining the two serum concentrations.*
- Goal serum trough concentration:

Drug	Goal 24-Hour Concentration (mcg/mL)
Gentamicin	<2
Tobramycin	<2
Amikacin	<6

- The typical dosing interval for patients on CRRT is every 24 to 48 hours.

IV.4.2   ADULT VANCOMYCIN PHARMACOKINETICS AND DOSING

Initial Dosing
- For patients with serious or life-threatening infections, a vancomycin loading dose of 25 mg/kg may be appropriate to ensure rapid attainment of target serum concentrations; maximum dose recommended as a single dose is 2,500–3,000 mg with an infusion rate of 1,000 mg/hr.
  - Consider a loading dose in critically ill patients with sepsis, patients with healthcare-associated pneumonia admitted to the ICU, or those patients who are critically ill with a strong suspicion for infection with MRSA, MRSE, or *Enterococcus* spp.
- Maintenance dose of 15–20 mg/kg; interval may be determined by patient-specific creatinine clearance (renal function should be completely considered [i.e., urine output, trends in SCr, fluid status, etc.])
- Dose should be based on actual body weight
  - If patient is obese, dose on actual body weight and adjust based on steady-state (prior to fourth dose) trough concentrations

Initial Vancomycin Dosing Table

Simplified Adult Vancomycin Dosing Algorithm Target Trough 10–20 mcg/mL A loading dose of 25–30 mg/kg × 1 (not to exceed a single dose of 2,500–3,000 mg) may be used in critically ill patients		
Creatinine Clearance (mL/min)	**Dosing Unit**	**Interval**
>50	15–20 mg/kg/ dose	Q12h – Q8h*†
20–49		Q24h
<20		Q24h × 2 doses, followed by level; repeat frequency dependent on renal function and level (usually Q48–72h)
Intermittent Hemodialysis		See IHD recommendations below
CRRT		See CRRT recommendations below

* Not to exceed more than 3,000–4,000 mg/day
† Consider initial Q8h dosing in patients <30 years of age, CrCl >80 mL/min, and/or ABW >100 kg with normal renal function

General Dosing Recommendations
- Dose is rounded to the nearest 250 mg
- The maximum rate of infusion is 1,000 mg per hour (the deliberately slow infusion is a strategy to prevent the risk of histamine-related infusion-related reactions, or Red Man Syndrome, marked by hypotension, flushing, and pruritis)
- Total daily doses >3,000–4,000 mg should be used with caution due to the risk of nephrotoxicity

Initial Monitoring
- Trough concentrations are utilized as they are a marker to predict efficacy (AUC/MIC ratio). Peak concentrations are NOT recommended.
- For patients with an estimated CrCl of ≥20 mL/min, trough is only drawn prior to the fourth dose (steady state). There is rarely a reason to draw a trough before the drug reaches steady state as this may either overestimate or underestimate the true concentration.
- For patients with an estimated CrCl <20 mL/min, draw a random level on day 3 (24 hours after the second dose).

Monitoring Frequency:
- A vancomycin level is NOT always needed. Trough concentrations are not needed if:
  - The expected duration of vancomycin use is ≤3 to 5 days and stable renal function.
- At least one steady state vancomycin trough concentration is required for patients on prolonged courses (>3 to 5 days).
  - Follow-up trough concentrations should be performed weekly if patient is hemodynamically stable. Clinical judgment should guide frequency of monitoring.
    - More frequent vancomycin trough concentrations may be required in critically ill patients such as:
      - Fluctuating renal function or fluid balance
      - Concomitant nephrotoxic agents

- Older patients receiving Q8h dosing
- Not responding to initial dosing regimen or are decompensating on current regimen

Target Trough Concentrations:

- Vancomycin trough concentrations of 10–20 mcg/mL are recommended to improve penetration, increase the probability of obtaining optimal target serum concentrations, and improve clinical outcomes.
- A minimum trough concentration of 10 mcg/mL is required to avoid the development of resistance.
  - For *S. aureus* with an MIC <1 mcg/mL, goal trough = 10–15 mcg/mL.
  - For *S. aureus* with an MIC = 1 mcg/mL or severe infections (e.g., endocarditis, osteomyelitis, meningitis, HAP/VAP), goal trough = 15–20 mcg/mL.
  - For *S. aureus* with an MIC >1 mcg/mL, consider an alternative therapy as the target AUC:MIC of >400 is unattainable.

Follow-Up Dosing and Monitoring

Dosage Adjustments, *level based:*

Reassess patient's clinical status and continued need for vancomycin therapy based on indication, available culture data, etc.

- Evaluate trough concentration
  - Reassess patient renal function (stable, worsening, improving, etc.), confirm appropriate dose range and documented administration times
  - Establish validity of trough concentration, assess nursing administration time, time elapsed from prior dose, and appropriateness of concentration
- If trough concentration is greater than or less than 10 mcg/mL to 15 mcg/mL, depending on target range and renal function, the following calculation may be used to determine new dose due to the linear pharmacokinetics of vancomycin:

$$\frac{\text{total daily dose (mg)}}{\text{measured trough}} = \frac{x^*}{\text{goal trough}}$$

x = new dose in mg (not to exceed more than 3,000–4,000 mg/day)

* It is not recommended to increase dose more than 50%

- If there is a continued need for vancomycin, re-evaluate the serum trough concentration by the fourth dose, but earlier if:
  - Patient is hemodynamically unstable or renal function is changing.
  - Dosing interval is >24 hours.

Monitoring for Toxicity:

Per IDSA/ASHP/SIDP consensus statement, vancomycin has little potential for nephrotoxicity or ototoxicity when used as monotherapy.

- Nephrotoxicity: Monitor for nephrotoxicity, especially if patient is concomitantly receiving nephrotoxins.
  - Serum creatinine monitoring frequency

- Evaluate serum creatinine at least every 3 to 5 days if patient is stable.
- Daily monitoring of serum creatinine is appropriate in patients who are hemodynamically unstable.
    - ○ The definition of nephrotoxicity can vary:
        - Generally defined as a minimum of 2 to 3 consecutive documented increases in serum creatinine levels:
            - Increase of 0.5 mg/dL (for patients with SCr WNL) or
            - Increase greater than 20% from baseline (especially for patients with abnormal baseline creatinine).
- Ototoxicity: Per the IDSA/ASHP/SIDP consensus statement, monitoring for ototoxicity is not recommended for patients receiving vancomycin monotherapy; however, if the patient is receiving concurrently agents with ototoxic potential, then monitoring should be considered.

Adult Vancomycin Dosing and Monitoring in Hemodialysis and Continuous Renal Replacement Therapy

Intermittent Hemodialysis:
Vancomycin dosing in intermittent hemodialysis (IHD) is dependent on the type of dialysis and dialysis membranes utilized. New membranes increase the clearance of higher molecular weight molecules such as vancomycin.

Initial IHD Vancomycin Dosing and Monitoring:
(Assuming mid-high flux)
- Two consecutive daily 15–20 mg/kg doses should be administered regardless of dialysis schedule; this ensures rapid target concentration attainment.
- Draw a random level prior to the next HD session.

Subsequent Doses:
- Subsequent doses depend on the method and frequency of dialysis.
- Patients should be redosed (usually 15 mg/kg) once random vancomycin concentrations are less than 10–20 mcg/mL.
- NOTE: Careful attention should be placed on the IHD schedule (e.g., some patients require an extra HD session or a less frequent schedule than the typical Monday-Wednesday-Friday or Tuesday-Thursday-Saturday schedule) with dose adjustments made accordingly.

Monitoring:
- Random vancomycin concentrations of 15–20 mcg/mL are recommended. See information above for further explanation.
- Monitor the IHD plan (i.e., in the case of a patient requiring an extra HD session, or less frequent IHD, etc.).

For patients receiving low-flux HD, less frequent dosing ~1–2 (15 mg/kg) doses per week is usually required. Dose based on levels and re-dose once random concentrations are less than 10–20 mcg/mL.

Continuous Renal Replacement Therapy (CRRT):
Drug clearance is highly dependent on the method of renal replacement, filter type, and flow rate. Appropriate dosing requires close monitoring of pharmacologic response, signs of adverse reactions due to drug accumulation, as well as drug concentrations in relation to target trough concentration. The following are general recommendations only (based on dialysate flow/ultrafiltration rates of 1–2 L/hr and minimal residual renal function) and should not supersede clinical judgment:

CVVH: Loading dose of 15–25 mg/kg, followed by 15 mg/kg every 24–48 hours
CVVHD: Loading dose of 15–25 mg/kg, 15 mg/kg every 24 hours
CVVHDF: Loading dose of 15–25 mg/kg, 15 mg/kg every 12 hours

Subsequent Doses:
Once a patient is started on CRRT, draw a random level 24 hours after the last dose. Re-dose when vancomycin concentration is less than 10–20 mcg/mL and the frequency should be based on that initial level.

REFERENCE

Rybak, M, Lomaestro B, Rotschafer JC, et al. Therapeutic monitoring of vancomycin in adult patients: A consensus review of the American Society of Health-System Pharmacists, the Infectious Diseases Society of America, and the Society of Infectious Diseases Pharmacists. *Am J Health-Syst Pharm.* 2009; 66:82–98.

PART V

What Antimicrobial Stewardship Interventions Can Be Made on Reassessment and What Needs to Be Monitored?

V.1 ANTIMICROBIAL STEWARDSHIP BASICS—WHERE TO START AND HOW TO MAINTAIN

V.1.1 RATIONALE FOR STEWARDSHIP

Antimicrobials have transformed medicine, making once lethal infections readily curable. The prompt initiation of antimicrobials has been shown to reduce morbidity and mortality especially in patients with sepsis. However, approximately 50% of all antimicrobials prescribed in acute care hospitals in the United States are unnecessary or inappropriate— oftentimes a direct result of a lack of de-escalation or discontinuation when a noninfectious source is identified. The result is a challenging balancing act between appropriate empiric therapy and antimicrobial stewardship (AMS) efforts.

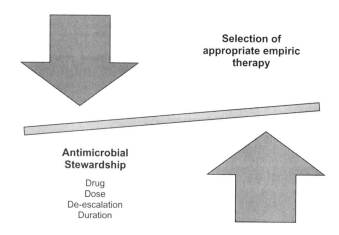

Selection of appropriate empiric therapy

Antimicrobial Stewardship

Drug
Dose
De-escalation
Duration

V.1.2 RISKS OF ANTIMICROBIAL MISUSE OR OVERUSE

Misuse and overuse of antimicrobials is associated with myriad consequences to not only individual patients but society as a whole. Some of these risks are listed below:
- Risk for serious adverse effects with no clinical benefit
  - Direct drug-related toxicity (e.g., nephrotoxicity from vancomycin or peripheral neuropathy from metronidazole, etc.)
  - Development of superinfections
    - *Clostridium difficile* infection
  - Patient-specific development of resistance
- Development of global resistance
  - Antimicrobial resistance is increasing and has become one of the most serious growing threats to public health and has significant detrimental effects on health care systems

○ Associated with increased risk of death, length of stay, and higher attributable costs
- Reduced number of antimicrobial agents approved in the past 25 years, with no clear recovery expected in the near future

V.1.3 PURPOSE AND GOALS

The purpose of AMS is to optimize safe, judicious, and appropriate use of antimicrobials, enhance clinical outcomes while minimizing unintended consequences of antimicrobial use, and reduce healthcare costs without adversely affecting quality of care. The primary focus of antimicrobial stewardship should be **patient safety**.

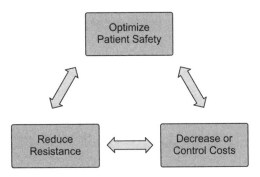

V.1.4 KEY AMS STAKEHOLDERS

The Infectious Diseases Society of America and Society for Healthcare Epidemiology of America *Guidelines for the Development of an Institutional AMS Program*[1] recommend a multidisciplinary group including co-leadership by an infectious diseases (ID) physician and ID-trained (or stewardship-trained) clinical pharmacist and include representation from hospital administration, infection prevention, information technology, microbiology, and front-line prescribers to initiate, track, maintain, and improve AMS efforts.

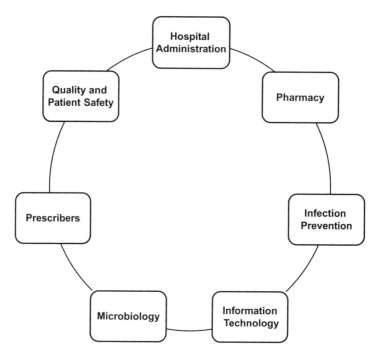

General AMS Stakeholder Roles

Hospital Administration Role: Formal supportive documents for AMS efforts, FTE designation for appropriate personnel to initiate, implement, and manage AMS efforts, and support ID or AMS training and education

Physician Leader Role: Responsible for AMS outcomes and assistance with development and implementation of AMS interventions

Pharmacy Role: Co-lead responsible for AMS outcomes, development, and implementation of AMS interventions, tracking, and reporting trends

Infection Prevention Role: Prevention, monitoring, and reporting hospital-acquired infections and resistance

Information Technology Role: Integration of electronic AMS efforts into practice (e.g., antimicrobial order sets, physician alerting, addition of clinical decision support tools)

Microbiology Role: Development and maintenance of hospital antibiogram, optimal use of laboratory testing, and result reporting

Prescribers Role: Engagement in and support of AMS efforts as antimicrobial prescribers

Quality and Patient Safety: Assistance with reporting and partnering with AMS team to optimize opportunities for improvement

V.1.5   SPECIFIC AMS INTERVENTIONS

As pharmacists, we are in the ideal role to intervene on AMS-related issues. In fact, many antimicrobial stewardship interventions can be made prior to patient receipt of any antimicrobial such as recommending appropriate first-dose empiric therapy based on empiric use guidelines and the institutional antibiogram, optimizing antimicrobial dosing based on patient-specific parameters, or perhaps recommending a watchful waiting period prior to the initiation of antimicrobials especially in the case of rhinosinusitis or bronchitis. It is oftentimes much easier to optimize therapy before a patient starts receiving antimicrobial therapy rather than once it has been initiated.

The following list provides information on suggested AMS interventions that can be implemented at a variety of institutions:

- *Essential information to include on all anti-infective orders*
  - **Drug**
    - Essential component of prescription
  - **Dose**
    - Essential component of prescription
    - Allows for optimization for specific situations such as renal insufficiency, resistant pathogens, etc.
  - **Indication**
    - Assists with dosing and therapeutic drug monitoring goals.
    - Is helpful to include whether the use is for empiric coverage, documented infection, surgical prophylaxis, or potentially medical prophylaxis (e.g., *Pneumocystis jiroveci* pneumonia prophylaxis, spontaneous bacterial peritonitis prophylaxis, *Mycobacterium avium* complex prophylaxis, etc.).
  - **Duration**
    - If duration can be tied to the indication, it may help prevent unnecessary prolonged duration of therapy.
    - For example, the default duration for empiric orders could be 72 hours with an alert to providers at the 48-hour time point that the patient's empiric therapy will be discontinued in 24 hours. Although daily assessment of empiric therapy is recommended, this allows for a reminder to take an antimicrobial "time-out" by reassessing the need for medications, making necessary changes in medications (such as increasing or decreasing the dose for renally dose-adjusted medications as appropriate, de-escalation of therapy based on culture data, or discontinuation of therapy based on identification of a noninfectious source of symptoms, etc.), or continuing empiric therapy (as is often the case for pneumonia). It is helpful for providers to take these actions directly through an electronic alert.
- *Development and implementation of evidence-based empiric anti-infective use guidelines*
  - Recommendations based on published guidelines for common infectious disease states (easily accessible via www.idsociety.org), local antibiogram, and formulary
    - E.g., central nervous system (CNS) infections, skin and soft tissue infections, pneumonia (community-acquired, healthcare-associated, hospital-acquired, ventilator-associated), intra-abdominal infections, urinary tract infections, *Clostridium difficile* infection (CDI), fungal infections, etc.
  - Include clinical decision support comments and tools for providers to guide therapy
  - Develop definitive infection guidelines including de-escalation recommendations
- *Formulary restriction*
  - Restriction either to a specific provider group or service or by indication (e.g., restricting daptomycin to ID physicians or requires ID physician or pharmacist approval prior to administration).

- Timeliness of antimicrobial administration is essential. Antimicrobials that are restricted should not be withheld if approval is anticipated to take time. Consider administering one dose until approval can be obtained (unless there is an appropriate alternative), especially in a patient with sepsis.

- *Prospective audit of antimicrobial use*
  - Review of antimicrobial use in specific hospital locations or by targeted antimicrobial agent (e.g., critically ill patients in the ICU, broad-spectrum, high-cost agents, restricted agents, etc.) with direct feedback and recommendations to providers.
  - Review of patients based on specific positive culture data from the laboratory
    — Especially those with positive blood cultures
    — Identification of drug-bug mismatches
  - Antimicrobial de-escalation based on cultures and clinical conditions:
    - Narrowing spectrum of activity
    - Discontinuation of duplicative or unnecessary therapy (e.g., discontinuation of MRSA coverage when MRSA infection has been ruled out, discontinuation of non-CDI-associated antimicrobials when CDI is identified)
    - Always continually assess patient response to therapy (i.e., monitor resolution of subjective symptoms and objective data such as WBC and temperature normalization, hemodynamic stability, etc.)
  - Continued dose optimization based on organ function (e.g., renal dosing adjustments, etc.)
  - Monitoring length of therapy and recommendations to providers for de-escalation or discontinuation
  - Systematically document all above recommendations

- *Automatic IV to PO conversions*
  - Anti-infectives with good oral bioavailability can be converted from IV to PO in specific circumstances
    - Agents with oral bioavailability >80%: azithromycin, ciprofloxacin, doxycycline, fluconazole, levofloxacin, linezolid, tedizolid, metronidazole, moxifloxacin, sulfamethoxazole/trimethoprim
    - Possible inclusion criteria:
      - Functioning GI tract
      - Receiving other oral medications
      - Tolerating diet
      - No nausea, vomiting, or profuse diarrhea
      - Patient is clinically stable
        - Absence of life-threatening infection (e.g., bacteremia, endocarditis, febrile neutropenia, meningitis, osteomyelitis, sepsis, or septic shock)
        - Patient has received IV therapy for at least 24 hours
        - Afebrile for >24 hours
        - Normalizing WBC
        - Stable vital signs (blood pressure, heart rate, respiratory rate)
      - Lack of aspiration risk

V.1.6   MONITORING AND REPORTING

Monitoring and measurement of impact is essential yet challenging to identify opportunities for improvement and to assess the efficacy or impact of implemented AMS interventions and initiatives.

- *Process measurement—assess impact of efforts to improve antimicrobial utilization*
  - ○ *Intermittent assessment of antimicrobial use*
    - ▪ Review of specific drugs (medication-use evaluation) for appropriateness of drug selection, doses, identify if de-escalation opportunities were optimized, duration, etc.
    - ▪ Review specific indications (e.g., community-acquired pneumonia, CDI)
    - ▪ Timeliness (especially for sepsis, severe sepsis, and septic shock)
    - ▪ Specific provider performance on antimicrobial utilization and quality of antimicrobial "time-outs" and re-assessments
    - ▪ Document interventions from the prospective audit and feedback process so as to assess acceptance
  - ○ *Measuring antimicrobial consumption*
    - ▪ Overall and unit-specific
      - ○ *Days of Therapy (DOT):* Aggregate sum of days for which any amount of a specific antimicrobial agent is administered or dispensed to a particular patient (numerator) divided by a standardized denominator (e.g., patient days, days present, or admissions).
        - — E.g., If a patient received 3 antimicrobials for 10 days, the DOT numerator would be 30.
        - — *DOT Advantages:* More applicable to different populations (adult and pediatric patients), less likely to be affected by different dosing schemes, more applicable to benchmarking.
        - — *DOT Limitations:* Renal function adjustments that require less than daily dosing results in inaccurate reflection of antimicrobial exposure.
      - ○ *Defined Daily Dose (DDD):* Estimates hospital antimicrobial use by aggregating the total number of grams of each antimicrobial purchased, dispensed, or administered during a period of time divided by the World Health Organization-assigned DDD (www.whocc.no).[2]
        - — WHO DDD data for antimicrobials are in grams or million units.
        - — E.g., If 4,000 mg of azithromycin was dispensed in one month, convert to 4 g, divide this by the WHO DDD of 0.5 g, then the DDD is 8. To then calculate DDD/1,000 patient days, determine the patient days for the unit in question or hospital overall for the same time period. If your ICU had 425 patient days, the DDD/1,000 patient days would be as follows: $8/425 \times 1,000 = 18.8$.
        - — *DDD Advantages:* May be useful progress measure if consistently tracked over time.
        - — *DDD Limitations:* Not appropriate for children or for patients with reduced drug excretion such as renal impairment and less reliable for benchmarking utilization.
      - ○ *Other*: drug acquisition data, dispensed prescriptions, medication orders, units purchased

> — *Advantage*: Easy to obtain
>
> — *Limitations*: Oftentimes inaccurate as there are many confounding variables such as different manufacturers/wholesalers in times of drug shortages affecting total drug counts; does not consider unused returned medications; and most significantly, does not reflect true patient consumption via actual administration.

- *Outcome measurement—assess impact of AMS interventions on clinical outcomes*
  - ○ *Track and trend clinical outcomes*
    - ▪ Resistance
  - ○ *Resistance trends*—should be monitored over time and assessed to assist with empiric use guidelines and modifications in the guidelines as necessary
  - ○ *Resistance as a sole marker of AMS efforts*—is limited as the development of resistance is multifactorial
  - ○ *Potentially tracking resistance development*—for specific patients after receipt of antimicrobials
    - ▪ CDI rates
    - ▪ Mortality and hospital and/or ICU length of stay for specific ID syndromes
  - ○ *Costs*—after implementation of AMS efforts, costs decline and savings stabilize
    - ▪ Unintended consequences
    - ▪ Drug acquisition

Resources

There are many software programs available for AMS purposes such as TheraDoc® and MedMined®. These can help to more readily capture DDD and/or DOT and more quickly identify targeted patients for AMS interventions with an alert-based approach. In addition, the CDC has developed a surveillance program for antimicrobial use called The Antimicrobial Use and Resistance Option (see www.cdc.gov/nhsn/acute-care-hospital/aur/ for more details), in which sites or health systems can electively enroll and report monthly antimicrobial consumption and resistance data through the use of their Electronic Medication Administration Record (eMAR) or Bar Coding Medication Administration (BCMA) systems through collaboration with an affiliated vendor.

V.1.7   AMS EDUCATION

AMS teams are a key educational resource for antimicrobial stewardship-related issues. There should be a well-defined process and format for the dissemination of antimicrobial prescribing updates, formulary changes, site-specific guidelines, and site and national antimicrobial resistance trends. This can be achieved in a variety of formats such as:

- AMS monthly or quarterly newsletters
- Didactic presentations to specific provider groups or hospital unit-specific personnel
- Electronic communication via email or messaging systems

- Devoted space on the institution's intranet homepage for AMS resources and communication
- Pocket cards for distribution with the most utilized or most relevant ID-related recommendations
- Site-specific AMS app development

Educational efforts tend to be most impactful when site-specific data can be simultaneously presented to highlight issues or areas for improvement including process and outcome measures.

A helpful resource for AMS promotion and initiatives is the Centers for Disease Control and Prevention Get Smart About Antibiotics website (www.cdc.gov/getsmart/week/). There are a number of activity and event recommendations, educational resources, and promotional materials targeted toward healthcare providers and patients available for download and distribution.

There are also two antimicrobial stewardship certificate programs with associated continuing education credit available for pharmacists: The Society of Infectious Diseases Pharmacists (SIDP) Antimicrobial Stewardship Certificate Program and the Making a Difference in Infectious Diseases (MAD-ID) Antimicrobial Stewardship Program.

The SIDP program is comprised of a combination of self-study modules (24 hours), live webinars (6–9 hours), and a skills component completed in the practice setting (10 hours). The cost is approximately $750; however, a group discount may be applied if at least six people from the same institution participate or for trainees such as residents, fellows, etc. More information can be found at www.sidp.org/page-1442823.

The MAD-ID program offers two separate tracks: the basic program and the advanced program. The basic program offers participants the skills necessary to develop an Antimicrobial Stewardship Program, while the advanced program is targeted toward pharmacists, physicians, and other providers with solid antimicrobial stewardship and general infectious diseases baseline knowledge. The basic program utilizes a similar combination approach as the SIDP program that covers basic concepts online (9 hours), live online programming (7 hours), and a practical component (3 hours). Whereas, the advanced program is delivered at the annual meeting with a practical component at the participant's practice site (total 15.5 hours of CE). More information can be found at www.mad-id.org/antimicrobial-stewardship-programs.

The combination of risk for adverse effects, increasing antimicrobial resistance, and decreasing novel antimicrobial approvals highlights the immediate need for AMS programs. *Start somewhere and measure your impact!*

REFERENCES

Dellit TH, Owens RC, McGowan JE, et al. Infectious Diseases Society of America and the Society for Healthcare Epidemiology of America Guidelines for developing an institutional program to enhance antimicrobial stewardship. *Clin Infect Dis.* 2007;44:159–77.

WHO Collaborating Centre for Drug Statistics Methodology. Available at www.whocc.no. Accessed in July 2015.

V.2   TOP 10 CLINICAL ANTIMICROBIAL STEWARDSHIP INTERVENTIONS/OPPORTUNITIES

1. Asymptomatic Bacteriuria

- Bacteria present in urine without the presence of UTI-related symptoms
- Does not require antimicrobial therapy with the exception of pregnant patients and patients undergoing a genitourinary surgical procedure
- Data suggest 45–65% of patients receive inappropriate antimicrobial therapy
- Unnecessary treatment does not decrease the incidence of symptomatic infection or improve outcomes
- Predisposes the patient to the development of resistance and other potential adverse effects

Potential Stewardship Interventions:

- Educational campaign highlighting the appropriateness of therapy (targeting specific provider groups or locations such as the ED, etc.)
  - Electronic reminders
  - In-services
  - Pocket cards
  - Newsletters, flyers
- Guidelines or clinical pathways with clinical decision support
- Pharmacist involvement on rounds with direct feedback to providers
- Daily review of positive urine culture data or commonly used UTI antimicrobial agents to identify opportunities for improvement and direct intervention
- Suppression of laboratory urine culture susceptibility data with a prompt to providers to call lab for susceptibilities in symptomatic patients

Suggested Reading

Chowdhury F, Sarkar K, Branche A, et al. Preventing the inappropriate treatment of asymptomatic bacteriuria at a community teaching hospital. *J Community Hosp Intern Med Perspect.* 2012;2:17814.

Leis JA, Rebick GW, Daneman N, et al. Reducing antimicrobial therapy for asymptomatic bacteriuria among non-catheterized inpatients: a proof-of-concept study. *Clin Infect Dis.* 2014;58:980–983.

Nicolle LE, Bradley S, Colgan R, et al. Guidelines for the diagnosis and treatment of asymptomatic bacteriuria in adults. *Clin Infect Dis.* 2005;40:643–654.

Pavese P, Saurel N, Labarere J, et al. Does an educational session with an infectious diseases physician reduce the use of inappropriate antibiotic therapy for inpatients with positive urine culture results? A controlled before-and-after study. *Infect Control Hosp Epidemiol.* 2009;30:596–599.

2. Bacteremia

- Blood cultures should be drawn prior to antimicrobial administration for any patient with high suspicion of bacteremia (or fungemia), which may include hospitalized patients with:
  - Fever and leukocytosis or leukopenia (NOTE: A normal WBC count does not rule out bacteremia.)
  - Hemodynamic instability of unknown etiology
  - Possible intravascular infection (i.e., catheter-associated bacteremia, endocarditis, etc.)

- Antimicrobial administration should not be delayed if blood cultures cannot be obtained
- Blood cultures are especially important in the following disease states: known or suspected sepsis, endocarditis, meningitis, osteomyelitis, peritonitis, pneumonia, fever of unknown origin
- At least two sets of blood cultures should be obtained from two separate sites
- Careful assessment when skin commensals such as *Micrococcus* spp., coagulase-negative *Staphylococcus*, gram-positive bacilli (e.g., *Corynebacterium* spp., *Bacillus* spp., diphtheroids, etc.) are isolated as contamination is likely
  - When commensal skin organisms cause actual infection, it is often related to an indwelling catheter or device
  - Consideration of the presence of intravascular catheters and other prosthetic material is warranted as well as the number of positive cultures and patient's clinical status
- *S. aureus*, most *Streptococcus* spp., gram-negative organisms, and yeast are *almost* NEVER contaminants
- Surveillance cultures should be performed 1–2 days after positive blood culture and initiation of antimicrobials to confirm clearance
- IV therapy is preferred in most cases
- Treatment duration varies and should be directed at the source (longer courses are required when associated endocarditis, osteomyelitis, etc.)

Potential Stewardship Interventions:

- Implementation of rapid diagnostic tests such as Matrix-Assisted Laser Desorption/Ionization Time-of-Flight Mass Spectrometry (MALDI-TOF) for timely organism identification with targeted antimicrobial stewardship recommendations
  - MALDI-TOF can reduce time to identification by 1.2–1.5 days compared with traditional practices
- Daily review of all patients with positive blood cultures
- Discontinuation of empiric vancomycin when skin commensals identified and determined to be contaminants
- ID Consult should be strongly considered in most cases, especially for *S. aureus* bacteremia
  - Mandatory ID consult has been associated with improved outcomes for patients with *S. aureus* bacteremia
    - 56% reduction in 28-day mortality
    - More frequent echocardiography (59% vs 26%, $p < 0.01$), vancomycin trough concentration measurements (99% vs 77%, $p < 0.01$), source control (83% vs 57%, $p = 0.03$), follow-up blood cultures (71% vs 50%, $p = 0.05$), longer duration of anti-MRSA therapy (median and IQR: 17 days, 13–30 vs 12, 3–14, $p < 0.01$) and a 20% reduction in 7-day, 30-day, and in-hospital mortality
- If transition to oral therapy is appropriate, antimicrobial drug selection should include a bactericidal agent with excellent oral bioavailability (e.g., urinary source with documented evidence of organism clearance from blood)
- Duration of therapy is variable based on site and severity of infection

○ Shorter courses (5–7 days) *versus* longer courses (7–21 days), excluding endocarditis, have been associated with similar outcomes (i.e., clinical and microbiologic cure rates and survival)

Suggested Reading

Havey TC, Fowler RA, Daneman N. Duration of antibiotic therapy for bacteremia: a systemic review and meta-analysis. *Crit Care.* 2011;15:R267.

Honda H, Krauss MJ, Jones JC, et al. The value of infectious diseases consultation in *Staphylococcus aureus* bacteremia. *Am J Med.* 2010;123:631–637.

Huang AM, Newton D, Kunapuli A, et al. Impact of rapid organism identification via matrix-assisted laser desorption/ionization time-of-flight combined with antimicrobial stewardship team intervention in adult patients with bacteremia and candidemia. *Clin Infect Dis.* 2013;57:1237–1245.

Nagel JL, Huang AM, Kunapuli A, et al. Impact of antimicrobial stewardship intervention on coagulase-negative Staphylococcus blood cultures in conjunction with rapid diagnostic testing. *J Clin Microbiol.* 2014;52:2849–2854.

Perez KK, Olsen RJ, Musick WL, et al. Integrating rapid pathogen identification and antimicrobial stewardship significantly decreases hospital costs. *Arch Pathol Lab Med.* 2013;137:1247–1254.

Tissot F, Calandra T, Prod'hom G, et al. Mandatory infectious diseases consultation for MRSA bacteremia is associated with reduced mortalilty. *J Infect.* 2014;69:226–234.

3. β-Lactam Allergies

- PCN is the most frequently reported cause of drug allergy (up to 5–10% of general population reporting an allergy)
  ○ 95% of patients who report PCN allergy are not truly allergic
- Cross-allergy is an area of debate for β-lactams
- Newer literature suggests <3% and <1% rates of cross-reactivity for cephalosporins and carbapenems, respectively, and no chance of cross-reactivity to monobactams
- Allergy over-reporting leads to use of less efficacious and more toxic antimicrobials that may also have a higher risk of resistance development such as aminoglycosides and aztreonam

Potential Stewardship Interventions:

- Incorporation of the following comprehensive allergy assessment items upon hospital admission or outpatient visit to clarify important details of the reaction is essential:
  ○ Specific drug responsible for reaction
  ○ Dosage form utilized when reaction occurred
  ○ Description of symptoms
  ○ Time course of reaction in relation to drug administration
  ○ Treatment required to manage reaction
  ○ Observation of reaction by healthcare provider
  ○ Date of reaction (>10 years prior)
  ○ Other antimicrobial exposure since reaction
- Potential implementation of penicillin skin testing to assess true allergy in specific patients
- Aztreonam restriction or specific use criteria
- Implementation of a β-lactam allergy guideline, including details about the different types of reactions and descriptions of antimicrobials that can safely be administered
  ○ E.g., third- and fourth-generation cephalosporins and carbapenems are safe to administer in patients with a documented IgE-mediated reaction to penicillin

Suggested Reading

Benninger MS. Cephalosporin use in treatment of patients with penicillin allergies. *J Am Pharm Assoc.* 2008;48:530.

Borch JE, Anderson KE, Bindslev-Jensen C. The prevalence of suspected and challenge-verified penicillin allergy in a university hospital population. *Basic Clin Pharmacol Toxicol.* 2006;98:357–362.

Campagna JD, Bond MC, Schabelman E, et al. The use of cephalosporins in penicillin-allergic patients: a literature review. *J Emerg Med.* 2012;42:612–620.

Frumin J, Gallagher JC. Allergic cross-sensitivity between penicillin, carbapenem, and monobactam antibiotics: what are the chances? *Ann Pharmacother.* 2009;43:304–315.

International Rheumatic Fever Study Group. Allergic reactions to long-term benzathine penicillin prophylaxis for rheumatic fever. International rheumatic fever study group. *Lancet.* 1991;337:1308–1310.

Novalbos A, Sastre J, Cuesta J, et al. Lack of allergic cross-reactivity to cephalosporins among patients allergic to penicillins. *Clin Exp Allergy.* 2001;31:438–443.

Rimawi RH, Cook PP, Gooch M, et al. The impact of penicillin skin testing on clinical practice and antimicrobial stewardship. *J Hosp Med.* 2013;8:341–345.

Solensky R. Allergy to beta-lactam antibiotics. *J Allergy Clin Immunol.* 2012;130;1442–2.e5.

Wong BBL, Keith PK, Waserman S. Clinical history as a predictor of penicillin skin test outcome. *Ann Allergy Asthma Immunol.* 2006;97:169–174.

4. Intra-Abdominal Infections

- Successful management of intra-abdominal infections involves a combination of adequate source control and appropriate antimicrobial therapy
- In the presence of adequate source control, the guidelines recommend 4–7 days of antimicrobials
  - Short course (4 days) *versus* longer course (8 days) has been associated with similar outcomes (i.e., incidence of surgical site infection, recurrent intra-abdominal infection, or death stressing the significance of adequate source control)
- Growth of yeast or *Enterococcus* spp. from intra-abdominal cultures does not always warrant treatment, especially if the patient is clinically improving
- For appendicitis without perforation or necrosis, 24 hours of broad-spectrum perioperative antimicrobials or a single perioperative dose may be sufficient
- For uncomplicated diverticulitis (no evidence of perforation or abscess), no antimicrobials are needed
- For pancreatitis, antimicrobial therapy should be reserved for severe cases involving confirmed infection of the pancreas via surgical intervention

Potential Stewardship Interventions:

- Review of patients receiving commonly utilized agents for intra-abdominal infections to identify opportunities for de-escalation or discontinuation of antimicrobial therapy after short course of therapy (and source control)
- Educational campaigns highlighting appropriate therapy (empiric, definitive, and avoidance of antimicrobial initiation in specific cases as above) as well as duration of therapy recommendations for intra-abdominal infections

Suggested Reading

Chabok A, Pahlman L, Hjern F, et al.; AVOD Study Group. Randomized clinical trial of antibiotics in acute uncomplicated diverticulitis. *Br J Surg.* 2012;99:532–539.

Daskalakis K, Juhlin C, Pahlman L. The use of pre- or postoperative antibiotics in surgery for appendicitis: a systematic review. *Scand J Surg.* 2014;103:14–20.

Mazeh H, Mizrahi I, Dior U, et al. Role of antibiotic therapy in mild acute calculus cholecystitis: a prospective randomized controlled trial. *World J Surg.* 2012;36:1750–1759.

Sawyer RG, Claridge JA, Nathens AB, et al. Trial of short-course antimicrobial therapy for intraabdominal infection. *N Engl J Med.* 2015;372:1996–2005.

Shabanzadeh DM1, Wille-Jorgensen P. Antibiotics for uncomplicated diverticulitis. *Cochrane Database Syst Rev.* 2012 Nov 14;11:CD009092.

Solomkin JS, Mazuski JE, Bradley JS, et al. Diagnosis and management of complicated intra-abdominal infection in adults and children: guidelines by the Surgical Infection Society and the Infectious Diseases Society of America. *Clin Infect Dis.* 2010;50:133–164.

5. Skin and Soft Tissue Infections (SSTIs)

- Consider purulent versus non-purulent SSTI (carbuncles, furuncles, abscesses *versus* cellulitis, erysipelas)
  - Purulent:
    - Mild, purulent SSTIs require only incision and drainage (I&D) to manage the infection (source control)—no antimicrobials are warranted in most cases
    - Short course of antimicrobials (5 days) indicated in moderate to severe, purulent SSTIs after I&D
    - When indicated, antimicrobials should target *S. aureus*
  - Non-purulent:
    - Oral antimicrobials targeting *Streptococcus* spp. indicated for mild infections
    - For moderate infections, IV antimicrobials targeting *Streptococcus* spp. indicated
    - For more severe infections, surgical evaluation necessary in addition to empiric broad-spectrum antimicrobial administration
    - Short course of antimicrobials preferred in mild to moderate cases (5 days)
- Diabetic foot infections (DFI)
  - Careful assessment of actual infection versus chronic wound is essential
  - Avoidance of antimicrobials in clinically uninfected wounds
  - Antimicrobials for infected DFI should be combined with appropriate wound care
  - Patients should be classified into mild, moderate, and severe categories based on symptoms
  - Therapy targeting aerobic gram-positive cocci in a patient with mild infection and no recent antimicrobial exposure is sufficient
  - Anti-pseudomonal therapy unnecessary except for patients with risk factors (e.g., residence in an area with a warm climate or history of infection with *Pseudomonas* spp.)
  - Anti-MRSA therapy indicated in patients with a history of MRSA infection, severe cases, or in area where local prevalence of MRSA infection or colonization is high
- Venous insufficiency-associated stasis dermatitis
  - May become acutely infected, thus warranting antimicrobials
  - Stable, chronic bilateral inflammation characterizing stasis dermatitis should not be treated with antimicrobials

Potential Stewardship Interventions:

- Educational campaigns stressing the role of I&D and avoidance of antimicrobial administration in mild, purulent SSTIs (this may be especially helpful in outpatient clinics and emergency departments [ED])

- Pharmacists in the ED are in the perfect position to assist with the avoidance of antimicrobials in these cases and recommend short courses (5 days) of antimicrobials when indicated
- Clinical electronic pathways, guidelines, or order sets providing real-time clinical decision support may help to guide appropriate therapy
- Daily review of specific patients/units or specific antimicrobial agents commonly misused for these indications to identify interventions (de-escalation, discontinuation, duration) and opportunities for improvement

Suggested Reading

Lipsky, BA, Berendt AR, Cornia PB, et al. 2012 Infectious Diseases Society of America clinical practice guideline for the diagnosis and treatment of diabetic foot infections. *Clin Infect Dis.* 2012;54:132–173.
Stevens DL, Bisno AL, Chambers HF, et al. Practice guidelines for the diagnosis and management of skin and soft tissue infections: 2014 update by the Infectious Diseases Society of America. *Clin Infect Dis.* 2014;59:e10–52.
Weingarten MS. State-of-the-art treatment of chronic venous disease. *Clin Infect Dis.* 2001;32:949–954.

6. Pneumonia

- Community-acquired pneumonia (CAP)
  - Warrants short course antimicrobial therapy (5 days)
  - Must rule out HF/COPD, etc. especially when the chest radiograph (CXR) is inconclusive (e.g., vascular congestion or edema, etc.)
  - Requires careful assessment of all factors such as patient's history, physical exam, WBC, sputum culture (if available), urine antigen tests, BNP, procalcitonin
  - If pneumonia deemed unlikely or a viral source has been identified, stop antimicrobials
  - No CXR to determine resolution of infection or duration of antimicrobials
- Healthcare-associated pneumonia (HCAP)
  - Once confirmed diagnosis, shorter duration preferred
  - Consideration for vancomycin use
    - Severity of illness (critically ill, ICU versus general medical floor)
    - Local prevalence of MRSA
    - If MRSA nasal and/or throat swab negative, consider discontinuation of empiric vancomycin
  - Short course of 7–8 days of therapy
    - 14 days if *Pseudomonas* spp., *Acinetobacter* spp., or other non-fermenting gram-negative bacilli

Potential Stewardship Interventions:

- Educational campaigns targeting appropriate diagnosis and treatment highlighting empiric and definitive therapy as well as appropriate duration
- Clinical electronic pathways, guidelines, or order sets providing real-time clinical decision support may help to guide appropriate therapy
- Implementation of rapid viral panels
- Daily review of specific patients/units or specific antimicrobial agents commonly used for pneumonia to identify interventions (de-escalation, discontinuation, duration)
- Inclusion of pharmacists on rounds on general medicine floors and ICUs to provide prospective review and audit with associated interventions

- Consider treatment received in hospital as part of the duration of therapy when performing medication reconciliation

Suggested Reading

American Thoracic Society, Infectious Diseases Society of America. Guidelines for the management of adults with hospital-acquired, ventilator-associated, and healthcare-associated pneumonia. *Am J Respir Crit Care Med.* 2005;171:388–416.

Boyce JM, Pop OF, Abreu-Lanfranco O, et al. A trial of discontinuation of empiric vancomycin therapy in patients with suspected methicillin-resistant *Staphylococcus aureus* health care-associated pneumonia. *Antimicrob Agents Chemother.* 2013;57:1163–1168.

Chaberny IF, Bindseil A, Sohr D, et al. A point-prevalence study for MRSA in a German University hospital to identify patients at risk and to evaluate an established admission screening procedure. *Infection.* 2008;36:526–532.

Ide L, Lootens J, Thibo P, et al. The nose is not the only relevant MRSA screening site. *Clin Microbiol Infect.* 2009;15:1192–1193.

Mandell LA, Wunderink RG, Anzueto A, et al. Infectious Diseases Society of America/American Thoracic Society consensus guidelines on the management of community-acquired pneumonia in adults. *Clin Infect Dis.* 2007;44:S27–72.

7. Otitis Media (OM)

- Viruses may be the cause in up to 45% of OM cases
- Observation off antimicrobials is recommended for certain cases

Age	Confirmed Diagnosis	Uncertain Diagnosis
<6 months	Antimicrobials recommended	Antimicrobials recommended
6 months to 2 years	Antimicrobials recommended	*Severe illness: antimicrobials recommended **Non-severe illness: observation
≥2 years	*Severe illness: antimicrobials recommended **Non-severe illness: observation	Observation
*Severe illness: moderate to severe ear pain or fever ≥102.6° F **Non-severe illness: mild ear pain and fever <102.6° F		

- Since guideline publication, two randomized, placebo-controlled trials supported early antimicrobial therapy for confirmed otitis media
- 62% reduction in treatment failure; 81% reduction for rescue therapy
- Earlier and more sustained resolution of symptoms with therapy

Potential Stewardship Interventions:

- Avoidance of antimicrobial therapy when viral sources are likely
- Appropriate, early-initiated antimicrobial therapy for patients with confirmed infection

Suggested Reading

American Academy of Pediatrics Subcommittee on Management of Acute Otitis Media. Diagnosis and management of acute otitis media. *Pediatrics.* 2004;113:1451–1465.

Hoberman A, Paradise JL, Rockette HE, et al. Treatment of acute otitis media under 2 years of age. *N Engl J Med.* 2011;364:105–115.

Tahtinen PA, Laine MK, Huovinen P, et al. A placebo-controlled trial of antimicrobial treatment for acute otitis media. *N Engl J Med.* 2011;364:116–126.

8. Acute Bronchitis

- Most cases are viral; however, acute exacerbations of chronic bronchitis may be bacterial
- Global Initiative for Chronic Obstructive Lung Disease (GOLD) guidelines recommend to treat when:
  - Dyspnea
  - Increased sputum volume
  - Increased sputum purulence
  - Systemic signs/symptoms of infection

Potential Stewardship Interventions:

- If antimicrobials are deemed necessary, use an abbreviated treatment course
  - 3-day as effective as a 10-day course (microbiologic success, symptom recovery, use of corticosteroids, duration of oxygen therapy, and length of stay)
- Broad-spectrum antimicrobials only indicated empirically if patient with recent history of resistant organisms and/or critically ill requiring mechanical ventilation

Suggested Reading

El Moussaoui R, Roede BM, Speelman P, et al. Short-course antibiotic treatment in acute exacerbation of chronic bronchitis and COPD: a meta-analysis of double-blind studies. *Thorax.* 2008;63:415–422.

Global Strategy for Diagnosis, Management, and Prevention of COPD, Global Initiative for Chronic Obstructive Lung Disease (GOLD) 2015. Available from: http://www.goldcopd.org/. Accessed June, 15, 2015.

Roede BM, Bresser P, El Moussaoui R, et al. Three vs. 10 days of amoxicillin-clavulanic acid for type 1 acute exacerbations of chronic obstructive pulmonary disease: a randomized, double-blind study. Clin Microbiol Infect. 2007;13:284–290.

Sethi S, Murphy TF. Infection in the pathogenesis and course of chronic obstructive pulmonary disease. N Engl J Med. 2008;359:2355–2365.

9. Acute Rhinosinusitis

- Most cases are viral and should not be treated with antimicrobials
- Most viruses and some bacterial infections resolve spontaneously within the first 7–10 days

Potential Stewardship Interventions:

- Consider antimicrobial therapy when:
  - Symptoms persist and patient is not improving in greater than or equal to 10 days
  - Patients have severe symptoms for greater than 3–4 days
  - Onset with worsening symptoms following a typical viral infection that lasted 5–6 days
- Counsel patients on symptomatic relief with nasal corticosteroids and saline irrigation as well as when to seek medical attention

- If antimicrobials are deemed necessary:
  - Amoxicillin for children
  - Amoxicillin/clavulanate for adults (doxycycline is an alternative to amoxicillin/clavulanate)
  - Duration: 5–7 days of therapy for adults and 10–14 days of therapy for children

Suggested Reading

Chow AW, Benninger MS, Brook I, et al. IDSA clinical practice guideline for acute bacterial rhinosinusitis in children and adults. *Clin Infect Dis.* 2012;54:e72–112.

Falagas ME, Karageorgopoulos DE, Grammatikos AP, et al. Effectiveness and safety of short vs. long duration of antibiotic therapy for acute bacterial sinusitis: a meta-analysis of randomized trials. *Br J Clin Pharmacol.* 2009; 67:161–171.

Gwaltney JM Jr, Wiesinger BA, Patrie JT. Acute community-acquired bacterial sinusitis: the value of antimicrobial treatment and the natural history. *Clin Infect Dis.* 2004; 38:227–233.

Hadley JA. Value of short-course antimicrobial therapy in acute bacterial rhinosinusitis. *Int J Antimicrob Agents.* 2005; 26(Suppl 3): S164–169.

Pichichero ME. Short course antibiotic therapy for respiratory infections: a review of the evidence. *Pediatr Infect Dis J.* 2000; 19:929–937.

10. Acute Pharyngitis

- Most cases are viral and should not be treated with antimicrobials
- 75% of adults who consult their physician for a sore throat receive antimicrobials
- Group A Streptococcus (GAS) is the only common cause of bacterial pharyngitis that warrants treatment with antimicrobials

Potential Stewardship Interventions:

- Rapid antigen detection testing reflexed to culture to confirm GAS
- Review of culture results and discontinuation of empiric antimicrobials for non-GAS causes of pharyngitis

Suggested Reading

Bisno AL. Acute pharyngitis: etiology and diagnosis. *Pediatrics.* 1996; 97:949–954.

Ebell MH, Smith MA, Barry HC, et al. The rational clinical examination. Does this patient have strep throat? *JAMA.* 2000; 284:2912–2918.

Linder JA, Stafford RS. Antibiotic treatment of adults with sore throat by community primary care physicians: a national survey, 1989-1999. *JAMA.* 2001;286:1181–1186.

Shulman ST, Bisno AL, Clegg HW, et al. Clinical practice guideline for the diagnosis and management of group A streptococcal pharyngitis: 2012 update by the Infectious Diseases Society of America. *Clin Infect Dis.* 2012:1–17.

V.3   RAPID DIAGNOSTIC TESTS FOR ANTIMICROBIAL STEWARDSHIP

Traditional organism identification and susceptibility can take up to 48–72 hours to finalize. Implementation of rapid diagnostic tests (RDTs) can significantly reduce time to organism identification by at least 24 hours compared with traditional methods. When combined with antimicrobial stewardship interventions, RDTs have been shown to:

Reduce
- Time to effective antimicrobial therapy
- Time to optimal antimicrobial therapy
- Overall antimicrobial utilization
- Hospital length of stay
- Mortality
- Hospital costs

Increase
- Clinical cure rates
- Likelihood of ID consultation

Summary of Available Rapid Diagnostic Tests for Antimicrobial Stewardship Initiatives

Assay	Specimen Source	Manufacturer/Brand	Detectable Organisms	Detectable Resistance Genes	Turnaround Time (h)
Matrix-Assisted Laser Desorption/Ionization Time-of-Flight Mass Spectrometry (MALDI-TOF)	All sites (blood, respiratory, urine, wound, etc.)	• Bruker MALDI Biotyper • BioMérieux/VITEK® MS System	Wide variety of organisms including bacteria and yeast	None	0.2–1
Multiplex PCR	Blood	• BD GeneOhm™ / StaphSR assay • Cepheid/Xpert® MRSA/SA and C. difficile/Epi assays • Biodiagnostics/ FilmArray blood culture identification (BCID)	• Acinetobacter baumannii • Candida spp. • Enterobacter cloacae complex • Enterococcus spp. • Escherichia coli • Haemophilus influenzae • Klebsiella spp. • Listeria monocytogenes • Neisseria meningitidis • Proteus spp. • Pseudomonas aeruginosa • Serratia marcescens • Staphylococcus spp. • Streptococcus spp.	• mecA • vanA • vanB • KPC	0.5–2
Nanoparticle Probe Technology (Nucleic Acid Extraction and PCR Amplification)	Blood	• Nanosphere/Verigene® blood culture gram-positive (BC-GP)	• Enterococcus faecalis • Enterococcus faecium • Listeria spp. • Staphylococcus aureus • Staphylococcus epidermidis • Staphylococcus lugdunensis • Streptococcus agalactiae • Streptococcus anginosus group • Streptococcus pneumoniae • Streptococcus pyogenes	• mecA • vanA • vanB	2.5

Method	Specimen	Test	Organisms	Genes	Time (h)
Nanoparticle Probe Technology (Nucleic Acid Extraction and PCR Amplification) (*Cont'd*)	Blood	• Nanosphere/Verigene® blood culture gram-negative (BC-GN)	• Acinetobacter spp. • Citrobacter spp. • E. coli • Enterobacter spp. • K. pneumoniae • K. oxytoca • Proteus spp. • Pseudomonas aeruginosa	• KPC • NDM • CTX-M • VIM • IMP • OXA	2.5
Peptide Nucleic Acid Fluorescent In Situ Hybridization (PNA FISH)	Blood	AdvanDx	• Candida albicans • Candida glabrata • Candida krusei • Candida parapsilosis • Candida tropicalis • Coagulase-negative Staphylococcus • E. coli • Enterococcus spp. • K. pneumoniae • Pseudomonas aeruginosa • S. aureus	• mecA	0.3–1.5
Polymerase Chain Reaction (PCR)	• Blood • Stool • Wounds	• Roche Molecular System/LightCycler® SeptiFast MecA • BD GeneOhm™/Cdiff assay • Cepheid/Xpert® C. difficile assay • Gen-Probe Prodesse/ProGastro Cd	• Clostridium difficile • S. aureus	mecA/SCCmec	1–6

Potential Stewardship Interventions:

- Work with the microbiologist to determine type of RDT to be implemented and decide on workflow (i.e., will the RDTs be continuously performed or in batches as this has an impact on timing, who will receive notification of the results, how will the results be delivered, etc.)
- Develop clinical pathways or guidelines clearly defining appropriate empiric therapy and definitive therapy based on identified organism(s)
- Educational campaigns targeting appropriate providers to disseminate RDT information and associated benefits in addition to guideline information
- Assess the impact on outcomes compared to baseline data as described above

Suggested Reading

Bauer KA, Perez KK, Forrest GN, et al. Review of rapid diagnostic tests used by antimicrobial stewardship programs. *Clin Infect Dis.* 2014;59:S134–145.

Bauer KA, West JE, Balada-Llasat JM, et al. An antimicrobial stewardship program's impact with rapid polymerase chain reaction methicillin-resistant *Staphylococcus aureus*/*S. aureus* blood culture test in patients with *S. aureus* bacteremia. *Clin Infect Dis.* 2010;51:1074–1080.

Clerc O, Prod'hom G, Vogne C, et al. Impact of matrix-assisted laser desorption ionization time-of-flight mass spectrometry on the clinical management of patients with gram-negative bacteremia: a prospective observational study. *Clin Infect Dis.* 2013;56:1101–1107.

Forrest GN, Mankes K, Jabra-Rizk MA, et al. Peptide nucleic acid fluorescence in situ hybridization-based identification of *Candida albicans* and its impact on mortality and antifungal therapy costs. *J Clin Microbiol.* 2006;44:3381–3383.

Forrest GN, Mehta S, Weekes E, et al. Impact of rapid in situ hybridization testing on coagulase-negative staphylococci positive blood cultures. *J Antimicrob Chemother.* 2006; 58:154–158.

Forrest GN, Roghmann MC, Toombs LS, et al. Peptide nucleic acid fluorescent in situ hybridization for hospital-acquired enterococcal bacteremia: delivering earlier effective antimicrobial therapy. *Antimicrob Agents Chemother.* 2008;52:3558–3563.

Goff DA, Jankowski C, Tenover FC. Using rapid diagnostic tests to optimize antimicrobial selection in antimicrobial stewardship programs. *Pharmacother.* 2012;32:677–687.

Heil EL, Daniels LM, Long DM, et al. Impact of a rapid peptide nucleic acid fluorescence in situ hybridization assay on treatment of Candida infections. *Am J Health-Syst Pharm.* 2012;69: 1910–1914.

Holtzman C, Whitney D, Barlam T, et al. Assessment of impact of peptide nucleic acid fluorescence in situ hybridization for rapid identification of coagulase-negative staphylococci in the absence of antimicrobial stewardship intervention. *J Clin Microbiol.* 2011;49:1581–1582.

Huang AM, Newton D, Kunapuli A, et al. Impact of rapid organism identification via matrix-assisted laser desorption/ionization time-of-flight combined with antimicrobial stewardship team intervention in adult patients with bacteremia and candidemia. *Clin Infect Dis.* 2013;57:1237–1245.

Ly T, Gulia J, Pyrgos V, et al. Impact upon clinical outcomes of translation of PNA FISH-generated laboratory data from the clinical microbiology bench to bedside in real time. *Ther Clin Risk Manag.* 2008;4:637–640.

Nagel JL, Huang AM, Kunapuli A, et al. Impact of antimicrobial stewardship intervention on coagulase-negative *Staphylococcus* blood cultures in conjunction with rapid diagnostic testing. *J Clin Microbiol.* 2014;52(8):2849–2854.

Parta M, Goebel M, Thomas J, et al. Impact of an assay that enables rapid determination of *Staphylococcus* species and their drug susceptibility on the treatment of patients with positive blood culture results. *Infect Contrc Hosp Epidemiol.* 2010;31:1043–1048.

Perez K, Olsen RJ, Musick WL, et al. Integrating rapid diagnostics and antimicrobial stewardship improves outcomes in patients with antibiotic-resistant gram-negative bacteremia. *J Infect.* 2014;69:216–225.

Perez KK, Olsen RJ, Musick WL, et al. Integrating rapid pathogen identification and antimicrobial stewardship significantly decreases hospital costs. *Arch Pathol Lab Med.* 2013;137:1247–1254.

Sango A, McCarter YS, Johnson D, et al. Stewardship approach for optimizing antimicrobial therapy through use of a rapid microarray assay on blood cultures positive for Enterococcus species. *J Clin Microbiol.* 2013;51:4008–4011.

Schweizer ML, Furuno JP, Harris AD, et al. Empiric antibiotic therapy for *Staphylococcus aureus* bacteremia may not reduce in-hospital mortality: a retrospective cohort study. *PLoS ONE.* 2010;5:e11432.

Terp S, Krishnadasan A, Bowen W, et al. Introduction of rapid methicillin-resistant *Staphylococcus aureus* polymerase chain reaction testing and antibiotic selection among hospitalized patients with purulent skin infections. *Clin Infect Dis.* 2014;58:e129–132.

Vlek AL, Bonten MJ, Boel CH. Direct matrix-assisted laser desorption ionization time-of-flight mass spectrometry improves appropriateness of antibiotic treatment of bacteremia. *PLoS ONE.* 2012;7(3):e32589.

Wong JR, Bauer KA, Mangino JE, et al. Antimicrobial stewardship pharmacist interventions for coagulase-negative staphylococci positive blood cultures using rapid polymerase chain reaction. *Ann Pharmacother.* 2012;46:1484–1490.

V.4   COMPARATIVE ESTIMATED DRUG ACQUISITION COST PER DOSE

Generic Name	Formulation	Cost per Dose		Typical Dosing Frequency (assumes normal renal function)	
Acyclovir	IV	500 mg	$$	IV: 5–10 mg/kg/dose Q8h (IBW)	
	PO	200 mg	$	PO: varies by indication 200–800 mg three to five times daily	
		400 mg	$		
		800 mg	$		
Amikacin	IV	500 mg	$$	Traditional	Extended interval
		1 g	$$	5–7.5 mg/kg/dose Q8h	15–20 mg/kg Q24h
Amoxicillin	PO	500 mg	$	500 mg Q8h	
		875 mg	$	875 mg Q12h	
Amoxicillin/clavulanate	PO	500/125 mg	$	500 mg Q8h	
		875/125 mg	$	875 mg Q12h	
Amphotericin B (conventional)	IV	50 mg	$$$	0.4–1 mg/kg/dose Q24h	
Amphotericin B Lipid Complex (Abelcet)	IV	100 mg	$$$$$	5 mg/kg/dose Q24h	
Amphotericin B Liposomal (Ambisome)	IV	50 mg	$$$$	3–5 mg/kg/dose Q24h	
Ampicillin	IV	1 g	$	IV: 1–2 g Q6h	
		2 g	$	PO: 500 mg Q6h	
	PO	500 mg	$		
Ampicillin/subbactam	IV	1.5 g	$	1.5–3 g Q6h	
		3 g	$		

Drug	Route	Dose	Cost	Dosing
Anidulafungin	IV	100 mg	$$$$	Varies by indication 100–200 mg load followed by 50–100 mg Q24h
Azithromycin	IV	500 mg	$	500 mg Q24h
	PO	500 mg	$	(500 mg × 1 then 250 mg Q24h)
Aztreonam	IV	1 g	$$$	1–2 g Q8h
		2 g	$$$$	
Caspofungin	IV	50 mg	$$$$$	70 mg × 1 then 50 mg Q24h
		70 mg		
Cefaclor	PO	500 mg	$	500 mg Q8h
Cefadroxil	PO	500 mg	$	500 mg Q12h
Cefazolin	IV	1 g	$	1–2 g Q8h
		2 g	$	
Cefdinir	PO	300 mg	$	600 mg Q24h
Cefditoren	PO	200 mg	$$	200–400 mg Q12h
		400 mg	$$	
Cefepime	IV	1 g	$ $	1–2 g Q8–12h
		2 g		
Cefixime	PO	400 mg	$$	400 mg Q24h
Cefotaxime	IV	1 g	$	1–2 g Q6–8h
		2 g		
Cefotetan	IV	1 g	$	1–2 g Q12h
		2 g		
Cefoxitin	IV	1 g	$$	1–2 g Q6h
		2 g	$$$	

(continued)

Generic Name	Formulation	Cost per Dose	Typical Dosing Frequency (assumes normal renal function)
Cefpodoxime	PO	100 mg / 200 mg	$ / $$	100–400 mg Q12h
Cefprozil	PO	250 mg / 500 mg	$ / $	250–500 mg Q12h
Ceftaroline	IV	600 mg	$$$$	600 mg Q12h
Ceftazidime	IV	1 g / 2 g	$$ / $$	1–2 g Q8h
Ceftazidime/avibactam	IV	2.5 g	$$$$$	2.5 g Q8h
Ceftolazane/tazobactam	IV	1.5 g	$$$$	1.5 g Q8h
Ceftibuten	PO	400 mg	$$$	400 mg Q24h
Ceftriaxone	IV	1 g / 2 g	$ / $	1–2 g Q12–24h (most often Q24h)
Cefuroxime	IV	1.5 g	$	IV: 1.5 g Q6h
	PO	500 mg	$	PO: 500 mg Q12h
Cephalexin	PO	500 mg	$	500 mg Q6h
Cidofovir	IV	375 mg	$$$$$	5 mg/kg/dose once weekly to every other week
Ciprofloxacin	IV	200 mg / 400 mg	$ / $	IV: 200–400 mg Q12h
	PO	500 mg / 750 mg	$ / $	PO: 250–750 mg Q12h (400 mg IV = 500 mg PO)
Clarithromycin	PO	500 mg	$	500 mg Q12h
Clindamycin	IV	600 mg / 900 mg	$$ / $$	IV: 600–900 mg Q8h
	PO	300 mg / 450 mg	$ / $	PO: 300–450 mg Q6–8h

Drug	Route	Amount	Cost	Dosing
Colistin	IV	150 mg	$$	1–2.5 mg/kg/dose Q12h
Dalbavancin	IV	500 mg	$$$$$	1,000 mg × 1 then 500 mg × 1 one week later
Daptomycin	IV	500 mg	$$$$$	4 or 6 mg/kg/dose Q24h
Dicloxacillin	PO	500 mg	$	500 mg Q6h
Doripenem	IV	500 mg	$$$	500 mg Q8h
Doxycycline	IV	100 mg	$$	100–200 mg Q12h
	PO	100 mg	$	
Ertapenem	IV	1 g	$$$$	1 g Q24h
Erythromycin	PO	500 mg	$$	500 mg Q6h
Famciclovir	PO	500 mg	$$	250–500 mg Q8h
Fluconazole	IV	200 mg	$$	100–800 mg Q24h
	PO	100 mg	$	
		200 mg	$	
Flucytosine	PO	500 mg	$$$$	50–150 mg/kg/day Q6h
Ganciclovir	IV	500 mg	$$$$$	Induction (I): 5 mg/kg/dose Q12h Maintenance (M): 5 mg/kg/dose Q24h
Gentamicin	IV	10 mg/mL 2 mL 40 mg/mL 2 mL	$ $	Traditional: 1–2.5 mg/kg/dose Extended interval: 4–7 mg/kg
Imipenem/cilastatin	IV	500 mg	$$	500–1,000 mg Q6h
Itraconazole	PO	100 mg caps 100 mg/10 mL soln (150 mL)	$$ $$$$$	200 mg Q8h × 3 days then 200 mg Q12h
Ketoconazole	PO	200 mg	$	200–400 mg Q24h
Levofloxacin	IV	500 mg 750 mg	$$ $$$	500–750 mg Q24h
	PO	500 mg 750 mg	$ $	

(continued)

Generic Name	Formulation		Cost per Dose	Typical Dosing Frequency (assumes normal renal function)
Linezolid	IV	600 mg	$$$$	600 mg Q12h
	PO	600 mg	$$$$	600 mg Q12h
Meropenem	IV	500 mg	$$	1–2 g Q8h
		1 g	$$	
Metronidazole	IV	500 mg	$	500 mg Q8h
	PO	500 mg	$	
Micafungin	IV	100 mg	$$$$	100 mg Q24h
Minocycline	IV	100 mg	$$$$	100–200 mg Q12h
	PO	100 mg	$	
Moxifloxacin	IV	400 mg	$$	400 mg Q24h
	PO	400 mg	$$$	
Nafcillin	IV	1 g	$$	1–2 g Q4–6h
		2 g	$$	
Nitrofurantoin	PO	100 mg	$	100 mg Q6–12h
Norfloxacin	PO	400 mg	$	400 mg Q12h
Ofloxacin	PO	400 mg	$	200–400 mg Q12h
Oritavancin	IV	400 mg	$$$$$$	1,200 mg single dose
Oseltamivir	PO	75 mg	$$	Treatment: 75 mg Q12h Prophylaxis: 75 mg Q24h
Oxacillin	IV	1 g	$$	1–2 g Q4–6h
		2 g	$$$	
Penicillin G	IV	5 million units	$$	1–4 million units Q4–6h
Penicillin VK	PO	500 mg	$	500 mg Q6h
Peramivir	IV	600 mg	$$$$$$	600 mg once

Drug	Route	Dose form	Cost	Dosing
Piperacillin/tazobactam	IV	3.375 g / 4.5 g	$$ / $$	3.375–4.5 g Q6–8h
Posaconazole	IV	300 mg	$$$$$	200–400 mg
	PO	100 mg tab / 200 mg/5 mL 123 mL soln	$$$$ / $$$$$	Dose and frequency varies by indication
Quinupristin/dalfopristin	IV	500 mg	$$$$$	7.5 mg/kg/dose Q8h
Streptomycin	IM	1 g	$$	1–2 g Q12–24h
Sulfamethoxazole/trimethoprim	IV	400/80/5 mL 10 mL	$	IV: 2.5–5 mg/kg/dose Q6–8h
	PO	800/160 mg	$	PO: 800/160 mg Q6–8h
Tedizolid	IV	200 mg	$$$$$	200 mg Q24h
	PO	200 mg	$$$$$	
Telavancin	IV	750 mg	$$$$$$	10 mg/kg/dose Q24h
Tetracycline	PO	250 mg / 500 mg	$ / $$	250–500 mg Q6h
Telithromycin	PO	400 mg	$$	800 mg Q24h
Ticarcillin/clavulanate	IV	3.1 g	$$	3.1 g Q6h
Tigecycline	IV	50 mg	$$$$	100 mg × 1 then 50 mg Q12h
Tobramycin	IV	80 mg / 1.2 g	$ / $$	Traditional: 1–2.5 mg/kg/dose Q8h; Extended interval: 4–7 mg/kg Q24h
Valacyclovir	PO	500 mg / 1 g	$ / $	1–2 g; Varies by indication
Valganciclovir	PO	450 mg	$$$	450–900 mg Q12–24h
Vancomycin	IV	1 g	$$	IV: 15–20 mg/kg/dose Q6–48h; Varies based on therapeutic drug monitoring and indication
	PO	125 mg caps / 50 mg/mL 210 mL soln	$$$ / $$$$	PO: 125–500 mg Q6h

(continued)

Generic Name	Formulation	Cost per Dose		Typical Dosing Frequency (assumes normal renal function)
Voriconazole	IV	200 mg	$$$$	IV: 6 mg/kg load Q12h × 2 followed by 4 mg/kg Q12h maintenance
	PO	50	$$	PO: 200–300 mg Q12h (varies by indication)
		200 mg	$$$	
Zanamivir	INH	5 mg	$/dose	2 INH Q12h (10 mg total)
			$$$$/treatment course	

$ = less than $5.00 $$ = $5.01–20.00 $$$ = $20.01–50.00 $$$$ = $50.01–150.00 $$$$$ = $150.01–350.00 $$$$$$ = greater than $350.01

Appendix A

ASHP Statement on the Pharmacist's Role in Antimicrobial Stewardship and Infection Prevention and Control

POSITION

The American Society of Health-System Pharmacists (ASHP) believes that pharmacists have a responsibility to take prominent roles in antimicrobial stewardship programs and participate in the infection prevention and control programs of health systems. This responsibility arises, in part, from pharmacists' understanding of and influence over antimicrobial use within the health system. Further, ASHP believes that the pharmacist's ability to effectively participate in antimicrobial stewardship and infection prevention and control efforts can be realized through clinical endeavors focused on proper antimicrobial utilization and membership on multidisciplinary work groups and committees within the health system. These efforts should contribute to the appropriate use of antimicrobials, ultimately resulting in successful therapeutic outcomes for patients with infectious diseases, and reduce the risk of infections for other patients and healthcare workers.

BACKGROUND

Antimicrobial stewardship is utilized in practice settings of health systems to improve patient outcomes while minimizing the unintended consequences of antimicrobial use. The goals of antimicrobial stewardship programs include attenuating or reversing antimicrobial resistance, preventing antimicrobial-related toxicity, and reducing the costs of inappropriate antimicrobial use and healthcare-associated infections. Guidelines published by the Infectious Diseases Society of America and the Society for Healthcare Epidemiology of America and endorsed by ASHP and other organizations describe an evidence-based approach to antimicrobial stewardship in health systems and the important role pharmacists with infectious diseases training have in leading stewardship efforts.[1]

Identifying and reducing the risks of developing, acquiring, and transmitting infections among patients, healthcare workers, and others are an important part of improving patient outcomes. In order to maximize outcomes, antimicrobial stewardship should be used in combination with infection prevention and control practices.[1] Most health systems maintain an infection prevention and control program directed by a multidisciplinary committee. The specific program and responsibilities of the infection prevention and control committee (or its equivalent) may differ among health systems.

Typically, the infection prevention and control committee develops organizational policies and procedures addressing

1. The management and provision of patient care and employee health services regarding infection or infection prevention and control.
2. The education of staff, patients, family members, and other caregivers in the prevention and control of infections.
3. Surveillance systems to track the occurrence and transmission of infections.
4. Surveillance systems to track the use of antimicrobials and the development of antimicrobial resistance.
5. Promotion of evidence-based practices and interventions to prevent the development of infections.

RESPONSIBILITIES OF PHARMACISTS

Pharmacists' responsibilities for antimicrobial stewardship and infection prevention and control include promoting the optimal use of antimicrobial agents, reducing the transmission of infections, and educating health professionals, patients, and the public.

Promoting Optimal Use of Antimicrobial Agents

An important clinical responsibility of the pharmacist is to ensure the optimal use of antimicrobial agents throughout the health system. Functions related to this responsibility may include

1. Encouraging multidisciplinary collaboration within the health system to ensure that the prophylactic, empirical, and therapeutic uses of antimicrobial agents result in optimal patient outcomes. These activities may include antimicrobial-related patient care (e.g., aiding in appropriate selection, optimal dosing, rapid initiation, and proper monitoring and de-escalation of antimicrobial therapies) as well as the development of restricted antimicrobial-use procedures, therapeutic interchange, treatment guidelines, and clinical care plans.[2]
2. Working within the pharmacy and therapeutics committee (or equivalent) structure, which may include infectious disease-related subcommittees, to ensure that the number and types of antimicrobial agents available are appropriate for the patient population served. Such decisions should be based on the needs of special patient populations and

microbiological trends within the health system. High priority should be given to developing antimicrobial-use policies that result in optimal therapeutic outcomes while minimizing the risk of the emergence of resistant strains of microorganisms.

3. Operating a multidisciplinary, concurrent antimicrobial stewardship program that uses patient outcomes to assess the effectiveness of antimicrobial use policies throughout the health system.
4. Generating and analyzing quantitative data on antimicrobial drug use to perform clinical and economic outcome analyses.
5. Working with the microbiology laboratory personnel to ensure that appropriate microbial susceptibility tests are reported on individual patients in a timely manner, and collaborating with the laboratory, infectious diseases specialists, and infection preventionists in compiling susceptibility reports (at least annually) for distribution to prescribers within the health system to guide empirical therapy.
6. Utilizing information technology to enhance antimicrobial stewardship through surveillance, utilization and outcome reporting, and the development of clinical decision-support tools.
7. Facilitating safe medication management practices for antimicrobial agents by utilizing efficient and effective systems to reduce potential errors and adverse drug events.

Reducing the Transmission of Infections

Pharmacists should participate in efforts to prevent or reduce the transmission of infections among patients, healthcare workers, and others within all of the health system's applicable practice settings. This may be accomplished through

1. Participating in the infection prevention and control committee (or its equivalent).
2. Establishing internal pharmacy policies, procedures, and quality-control programs to prevent contamination of drug products prepared in or dispensed by the pharmacy department. This is of paramount importance in the preparation and handling of sterile products.[3] Other considerations include (but are not limited to) provisions for cleaning pharmaceutical equipment (e.g., laminar-airflow hoods and bulk-compounding equipment) and establishment of appropriate personnel policies (e.g., limiting the activities of staff members who exhibit symptoms of a viral respiratory illness or other infectious condition).
3. Encouraging the use of single-dose packages of sterile drug products rather than multiple-dose containers, except in sterile environments.
4. Recommending proper labeling, dating, and storage of sterile products and multiple-dose sterile-product containers (if used).
5. Encouraging routine immunization (e.g., influenza vaccination) of hospital staff and others who impact the patient care environment, and promoting periodic screening for selected transmissible diseases (e.g., tuberculosis) in accordance with health-system policy and federal, state, or local regulations.
6. Promoting adherence to standard precautions by healthcare workers, patients, and others who impact the patient care environment.[4]
7. Collaborating in the development of guidelines for risk assessment, treatment, and monitoring of patients and healthcare workers who have been in contact with persons with a transmissible infectious disease.

8. Striving for zero tolerance of healthcare-associated infections, including surgical site infections, catheter-associated bloodstream infections, catheter-associated urinary tract infections, and ventilator-associated pneumonia.

Educational Activities

The pharmacist's role includes providing education and information about antimicrobial stewardship and infection prevention and control to health professionals, patients, and members of the public who come in contact with the health system's practice settings. Incorporating active intervention techniques, such as formulary restriction and preauthorization, enhances the effectiveness of educational activities in the patient care setting.[1] Specific activities may include

1. Providing clinical conferences, newsletters, and other types of educational forums for health professionals on topics such as antimicrobial use and resistance, decontaminating agents (disinfectants, antiseptics, and sterilants), aseptic technique and procedures, and sterilization methods.
2. Educating and counseling inpatients, ambulatory care patients, home care patients, and their families and caregivers in the following areas: adherence to prescribed directions for antimicrobial use, storage and handling of medications and administration devices, and other infection prevention and control procedures (e.g., medical waste disposal).
3. Participating in public health education and awareness programs aimed at controlling the spread of infectious diseases by
   a. Promoting prudent use of antimicrobials,
   b. Providing immunization access for children and adults, and
   c. Promoting appropriate infection prevention and control measures (e.g., proper hand hygiene techniques).
4. Providing exposure to antimicrobial stewardship and infection prevention and control practices through experiential and didactic training for practicing health-system pharmacists, students, residents, and research fellows.

EDUCATION AND TRAINING OF PHARMACISTS

ASHP recognizes that the current shortage of pharmacists with advanced training in infectious diseases and the limited number of training opportunities may require pharmacists without such training to assume some of the responsibilities described above. ASHP supports the expansion of pharmacy education and postgraduate residency training on infectious diseases in order to develop an adequate supply of pharmacists trained to deliver these essential services.

CONCLUSION

ASHP believes that pharmacists have a responsibility to take prominent roles in antimicrobial stewardship and infection prevention and control programs in health systems. Pharmacists should participate in antimicrobial stewardship and infection prevention an control efforts through clinical endeavors focused on proper antimicrobial utilization and membership on relevant multidisciplinary work groups and committees within the health system.

REFERENCES

1. Dellit TH, Owens RC, McGowen JE, et al. Infectious Diseases Society of America and the Society for Healthcare Epidemiology of America guidelines for developing an institutional program to enhance antimicrobial stewardship. *Clin Infect Dis.* 2007; 44:159–77.
2. American Society of Health-System Pharmacists. ASHP guidelines on the pharmacist's role in the development, implementation, and assessment of critical pathways. *Am J Health-Syst Pharm.* 2004; 61:939–45.
3. American Society of Health-System Pharmacists. ASHP guidelines on quality assurance for pharmacy-prepared sterile products. *Am J Health-Syst Pharm.* 2000; 57:1150–69.
4. Siegel JD, Rhinehart E, Jackson M, et al. 2007 guideline for isolation precautions: preventing transmission of infectious agents in healthcare settings, June 2007. www. cdc.gov/ncidod/dhqp/pdf/guidelines/Isolation2007.pdf (accessed 2009 Feb 18).

SUGGESTED READING

Centers for Disease Control and Prevention. Guideline for disinfection and sterilization in healthcare facilities, 2008. Accessed 15 December 2008. www.cdc.gov/ncidod/dhqp/pdf/guidelines/Disinfection_Nov_2008. pdf.

Centers for Disease Control and Prevention [CDC]. Guidelines for environmental infection control in health-care facilities: recommendations of CDC and the Healthcare Infection Control Practices Advisory Committee (HICPAC). *MMWR.* 2003; 52(No. RR-10):1–48.

Diekema DJ, Doebbeling BN. Employee health and infection control. *Infect Control Hosp Epidemiol.* 1995; 16:292–301.

Gardner P, Schaffner W. Immunization of adults. *N Engl J Med.* 1993; 328:1252–8.

Goldmann DA, Weinstein RA, Wenzel RP, et al. Strategies to prevent and control the emergence and spread of antimicrobial-resistant microorganisms in hospitals. A challenge to hospital leadership. *JAMA.* 1996; 275:234–40.

Kollef M, Shapiro S, Fraser, V, et al. A randomized trial of ventilator circuit changes. *Ann Intern Med.* 1995; 123:168–74.

MacDougall C, Polk RE. Antimicrobial stewardship programs in healthcare systems. *Clin Microbiol Rev.* 2005 Oct;18(4):638–56.

Sepkowitz KA. Occupationally acquired infections in healthcare workers. *Ann Intern Med.* 1996; 125:826–34,917–28.

Shlaes DM, Gerding DN, John JF Jr., et al. SHEA and IDSA Joint Committee on the Prevention of Antimicrobial Resistance: guidelines for the prevention of antimicrobial resistance in hospitals. *Clin Infect Dis.* 1997; 25:584–99.

This statement was reviewed in 2013 by the Council on Pharmacy Practice and by the Board of Directors and was found to still be appropriate.

Approved by the ASHP Board of Directors on April 17, 2009, and by the ASHP House of Delegates on June 16, 2009. Developed through the ASHP Council on Pharmacy Practice. This statement supersedes the ASHP Statement on the Pharmacist's Role in Infection Control dated June 3, 1998.

Curtis D. Collins, Pharm.D., M.S., is gratefully acknowledged for drafting this statement.

The bibliographic citation for this document is as follows: ASHP Statement on the Pharmacist's Role in Antimicrobial Stewardship and Infection Prevention and Control. *Am J Health-Syst Pharm.* 2010; 67:575–7.

Index of Drugs

Generic names appear in lower case italics, but brand names appear in upper case (first letter). Combination drug entries are hyphenated in addition to the individual drugs being listed separately. Drug class entries are noted with an asterisk (*).

A

Abelcet, 39, 166
acetaminophen, 58, 60, 108
acitretin, 148
acyclovir, 30, 152, 154, 156, 166, 210
afluzosin, 95
alprazolam, 95
allopurinol, 142, 143
amantadine, 157, 158, 160, 166
AmBisome, 39, 104, 166
amikacin, 5, 18, 30, 38, 67, 110, 111, 166, 177, 179, 180, 181, 182, 210
amiloride, 148
*aminoglycosides, 5, 16, 17, 18, 19, 28, 29, 30, 54, 62, 67, 72, 106, 110, 112, 154, 176, 177, 179, 180, 198
para-aminobenzoic acid, 147
aminopenicillin, 139, 140, 142
amiodarone, 95, 136
amoxicillin, 15, 19, 20, 22, 56, 58, 59, 60, 61, 63, 64, 68, 69, 81, 88, 89, 90, 139, 141, 142, 143, 164, 166, 203, 210
amoxicillin-clavulanate, 19, 20, 22, 56, 58, 61, 63, 64, 68, 69, 81, 142, 166, 203, 210
amoxicillin-clavulanic acid, 139
amodiaquine, 95
amphotericin B, 30, 32, 33, 34, 35, 154, 166, 210
amphotericin B colloidal dispersion, 104, 106, 108
amphotericin B deoxycholate, 104, 106, 108
amphotericin B-lipid complex, 39, 104, 106, 108, 166, 210

liposomal amphotericin B, 32, 33, 34, 35, 39, 104, 106, 108, 166, 210
ampicillin, 16, 17, 18, 19, 20, 22, 28, 29, 30, 37, 38, 45, 46, 48, 51, 62, 64, 69, 72, 81, 82, 89, 90, 139, 143, 164, 167, 210
ampicillin-sulbactam, 18, 22, 38, 45, 51, 62, 69, 72, 81, 82, 139, 167, 210
anidulafungin, 50, 52, 101, 102, 167, 211
*antacids, 95, 96, 97, 124
*antiarrhythmic agents, 123, 133
*antidepressants, tricyclic, 138
*antipsychotic agents, 158
*antivirals, 151, 157
astemizole, 95
atorvastatin, 95
avibactam, 19, 117, 118, 121, 168, 212
azithromycin, 15, 18, 21, 22, 58, 59, 60, 61, 63, 64, 65, 132, 133, 167, 192, 211
aztreonam, 5, 17, 18, 19, 29, 30, 37, 51, 52, 56, 62, 67, 72, 88, 89, 134, 164, 167, 198, 211
*azoles, 32, 92

B

*barbiturates, 95, 136
benzoyl peroxide, 80
bepridil, 95
bosutinib, 95
botulinum immunoglobulin, 21
buspirone, 138
busulfan, 136